Register Now for Online Access to Your Book!

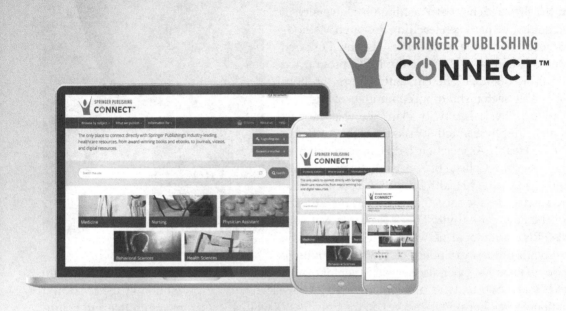

Your print purchase of *Research Methods for Public Health* **includes online access to the contents of your book**—increasing accessibility, portability, and searchability!

Access today at:
http://connect.springerpub.com/content/book/978-0-8261-8206-7
or scan the QR code at the right with your smartphone
and enter the access code below.

MGKLM1A1

D1157189

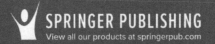

SPRINGER PUBLISHING
View all our products at springerpub.com

Amy A. Eyler, PhD, CHES, is an associate professor in the graduate program of public health in the Brown School at Washington University in St. Louis. She has been teaching Research Methods for over a decade and serves as the Research Methods course master for the MPH program at the Brown School. She currently chairs the public health sector standing committee of the U.S. National Physical Activity Plan. She was the past chair of the physical activity section of the American Public Health Association (APHA), a member of the American College of Sports Medicine (ACSM), and is a Certified Health Education Specialist. For over a decade, she served as principal investigator for the Physical Activity Policy Research Network (PAPRN), a national network of researchers who study the influence of policy on physical activity of a population. 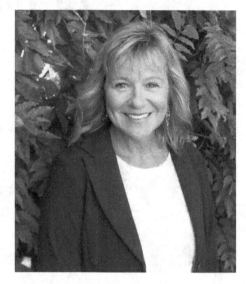 Dr. Eyler also served as senior associate editor for the *Journal of Physical Activity and Health*. She remains actively involved in physical activity promotion at the local and national level. Locally, she serves on the university's wellness steering committee and volunteers with several community organizations such as TrailNet and Girls on the Run. She has an extensive publication record, including the 2016 book *Prevention, Policy, and Public Health* and *Physical Activity and Public Health Practice* in 2019. She also contributed to the Institute of Medicine report *Educating the Student Body* and the 2017 U.S. National Physical Activity Plan Walking and Walkability Report Card. Dr. Eyler's main research interests are health promotion through community policy and environmental interventions, with a focus on physical activity and obesity prevention. She is a Faculty Fellow for Gender Equity, the president of the Association for Women Faculty, and a member of the University Faculty Senate Council. She has a master's degree in physical education and adult fitness from Ohio University and a doctorate in public health from Oregon State University.

Research Methods for Public Health

Amy A. Eyler, PhD, CHES

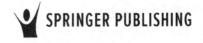

Springer Publishing Company, LLC
11 West 42nd Street, New York, NY 10036
www.springerpub.com
connect.springerpub.com/

Acquisitions Editor: David D'Addona
Compositor: diacriTech

ISBN: 978-0-8261-8205-0
ebook ISBN: 978-0-8261-8206-7
DOI: 10.1891/9780826182067

Qualified instructors may request supplements by emailing textbook@springerpub.com

Instructor's Manual ISBN: 978-0-8261-8207-4
Instructor's Test Bank ISBN: 978-0-8261-8208-1
Instructor's PowerPoints ISBN: 978-0-8261-8209-8
Instructor's Sample Syllabus ISBN: 978-0-8261-8211-1

22 23 24 25 26 / 6 5 4 3 2

The author and the publisher of this Work have made every effort to use sources believed to be reliable to provide information that is accurate and compatible with the standards generally accepted at the time of publication. The author and publisher shall not be liable for any special, consequential, or exemplary damages resulting, in whole or in part, from the readers' use of, or reliance on, the information contained in this book. The publisher has no responsibility for the persistence or accuracy of URLs for external or third-party Internet websites referred to in this publication and does not guarantee that any content on such websites is, or will remain, accurate or appropriate.

Library of Congress Cataloging-in-Publication Data
Library of Congress Control Number: 2020945662

Amy Eyler: https://orcid.org/0000-0001-8417-1656

Publisher's Note: **New and used products purchased from third-party sellers are not guaranteed for quality, authenticity, or access to any included digital components.**

Printed in the United States of America by Hatteras, Inc.

Contents

Preface

This book is truly a labor of love for me. I wanted to type "and now the fun begins" at the beginning of every chapter because I really think research *is* fun. The information is based on my experience teaching research methods to public health and social work students over the past decade and from my own academic research career. Research Methods is my absolute favorite course to teach. I get the opportunity not only to convince students of the importance of research, but also to build their skills and confidence in actually applying what they learn. No matter what background students come from, or what their public health career goals might be, research skills come in handy. Even if they never intend to conduct research studies after they graduate, they will at least be able to critically analyze studies for quality and merit. Research skills also help students to be good consumers of health information. We are inundated with claims about what is good for—or bad for—our health. Knowing how quality research studies are conducted and reported can help students believe or dispute the claims.

I have spent my entire academic career conducting public health research, particularly research related to chronic disease prevention through diet and physical activity. As a research professor, my livelihood was dependent on my ability to get grant funding, collect quality public health evidence, and make sure people knew about what I was doing. I had no choice but to be a successful researcher! The years of research experience provided me with knowledge that I pass along to students and now present in this book. Many of the examples and stories come from my own experiences and lessons learned.

Over the last decade, I have used several different textbooks in my classes. There were no books specific to public health, despite volumes for psychology, sociology, medicine, and social work. I started piecing chapters and readings together to create relevant course information for my public health students. Over time, I realized the type of information students need to build basic research skills and the best ways to present this information in class. This book is a compilation of over a decade of pilot testing.

I present information on research methods in a way that is complementary to other public health coursework. Epidemiology digs deep into specific methods for identifying distribution and determinants of health issues. An understanding of basic research methods serves as a foundation for mastery of epidemiology. Biostatistics is another component of public health preparation. The basic statistical concepts covered in research methods can supplement more advanced learning. In addition, skills such as efficiently reading and understanding research articles come in handy for many classes in undergraduate and graduate study.

This book is unique in many ways. First, each chapter aligns with the Council on Education for Public Health (CEPH) Master of Public Health Competencies. These competencies were recently revised, and accredited programs have to demonstrate how their courses prepare students to meet them. New to the competencies are skills such as budgeting and emphasis is placed on translating evidence and communicating public health information. With this in mind, an entire chapter is dedicated to research funding and budgeting, and two chapters—one on summarizing and visualization and another on dissemination—highlight the importance of not only conducting the research, but letting a broad audience know about it. For many public health professionals, these skills are lacking. It is my hope that with the required preparation, today's students will be well suited to effectively disseminate their work. Another unique feature of this book is its broad coverage of qualitative research. The updated CEPH competencies also require students to have qualitative (as well as quantitative) skills. Three chapters are dedicated to qualitative study design, data collection, and analysis.

Even though the topic of each chapter could fill an entire book, the material presented is thorough, yet concise. Each chapter provides enough information for students to confidently plan and conduct a basic research project, often a requirement of research methods courses. Additional resources and examples are provided throughout the book to help guide students through their own research exploration. The chapters also include ancillary information and examples relevant to each topic.

I am grateful to have the opportunity to share my experiences on every page of this book and I have many people to thank for their support and assistance. First, thank you to all of my research methods students, who helped me refine the information and method of delivery. I am thankful they endured my enthusiasm for research for semesters at a time! I am also thankful to countless mentors and supporters of my various research projects throughout the years, especially those within the Prevention Research Center of St. Louis. I had excellent reviewing and editing assistance from my colleagues Dr. Alan Beck and Ms. Rebekah Jacob. I also had help with graphics and figure design from Mr. Benjamin Volk, and I am thankful for his skills. I would also like to express my appreciation for my husband, Scott, and two children, Gabbie and Brad, for their love and support, and for putting up with me during the writing process.

Amy A. Eyler

PUBLIC HEALTH RESEARCH BASICS

This section provides the foundation for public health research methods. Chapter 1, The Importance of Research in Public Health, outlines the significance of research knowledge to students or practitioners of public health. This chapter also defines the steps in the research process, which are explained in detail in subsequent chapters. Chapter 2, Literature Search and Research Question Development, explains how a research question frames a public health study. It also outlines the significance of a literature review and provides some guidance on the literature review process. In Chapter 3, Ethics in Public Health Research, the history of public health research ethics is presented and described as the basis of current ethics policies. This chapter also explains the framework and guidelines for ethics in public health.

The Importance of Research in Public Health

Research is formalized curiosity. It is poking and prying with a purpose.

—Zora Neale Hurston, author

LEARNING OBJECTIVES

After reading this chapter, the reader will be able to

- Recognize the important role of research in public health.
- Understand the connection between research and evidence.
- Describe how evidence is created.
- Assess the quality of published research.
- Explain the steps in the research process.

INTRODUCTION

Research is both a process and an outcome. If you look up the word *research* in a dictionary, you will see it defined it as both a verb and a noun. We research topics through systematic investigation, but also use research as a source of facts and conclusions. Both of these descriptions are especially important in the field of public health. Research studies gather important information about behaviors, risk factors, and disease trends. Research also informs the development and testing of interventions for promoting health and preventing disease. The information gained from research can be used for advocacy efforts and to justify public health spending. Research might even be the catalyst for well, . . . more research! A single

TABLE 1.1 EXAMPLES OF DIFFERENCES IN DISEASE AND BEHAVIOR PREVALENCE, 2018

	Black (%)	White (%)	Urban (%)	Rural (%)	Less than HS (%)	College Grad (%)
Hypertension	41.1	34.0	45.1	47.0	42.6	27.8
Obesity	39.0	29.3	30.3	34.8	37.4	23.3
Diabetes	14.3	10.1	16.6	17.2	19.1	7.3
Smoking	18.5	17.1	12.4	18.2	27.3	6.5
Physical inactivity	32.2	25.0	28.9	33.8	44.2	15.5

HS, high school.

Source: United Health Foundation. American health rankings. 2018.
https://www.americashealthrankings.org.[3]

study rarely results in a definitive answer. "This topic warrants further study" is a common sentence written into conclusions of published research papers.

There have been tremendous achievements in public health over the last century, but many challenges to population health still exist. For example, the rates of communicable diseases have been quelled by improved sanitation and vaccinations, yet there is a staggering increase in the burden of preventable chronic diseases. According to the Centers for Disease Control and Prevention (CDC), one in six U.S. adults has at least one chronic disease,[1] and rates are predicted to rise. One reason for the projected increase is that risk of many chronic diseases increases with age. The U.S. Census Bureau estimates people 65 and older will comprise nearly 25% of the population by 2060.[2] There is a need for more research to plan for and address the health implications of this demographic shift. In addition, rates of chronic diseases vary greatly by factors such as race/ethnicity or geography (Table 1.1). Public health research is needed to identify ways to effectively reduce health disparities and create health equity.

Health equity means everyone has an equal opportunity for good health. Factors, such as poverty, lack of access to quality housing, education, and healthcare, impact the opportunity to live a healthy life and need to be addressed for health equity to exist.[4]

Lifestyle risk factors, such tobacco use, poor nutrition, lack of physical activity, and alcohol use, have tremendous impact on health and well-being.[1] It may seem as if some topics, such as tobacco use, are well researched and may not need additional study. After all, more than 7,000 studies were used to create the first report on smoking and health published in 1964,[5] over 50 years ago. Today, a quick literature database search on "smoking and health" results in a list of over 125,000 published articles; however, societal shifts and new trends warrant continued research. For example, electronic cigarettes were first introduced in the United States in 2006. Some recent research shows benefits of use in adults attempting to quit smoking traditional cigarettes, but long-term outcomes are unknown.[6] e-Cigarette use among adolescents is a recent public health concern. There is an increase in use among this population, and teens who use e-cigarettes are more likely to become tobacco smokers.[7] Research on prevention and cessation programs in this population is needed. Another current research gap is related to tobacco policies. Clean air policies, once only applicable to cigarette smoke, now are challenged to include e-cigarettes. Public health topics evolve and change over time, as does the need for research.

Technological advancements often create the need for new research. In the past, physical activity was assessed through self-report or direct observation of the behavior. Today, wearable fitness trackers and associated smartphone apps make activity easier to quantify, but studies are needed to understand the best ways to apply the data from these trackers to research.[8] The Internet provides a delivery method for interventions, increasing access to, for example, disease-prevention programs. Early studies show an evidence-based diabetes-prevention program (DPP) can be effective when implemented in an online format, but more research is needed to confirm its effectiveness across populations.[9] In addition, the ways in which internet use (e.g., social media) impacts health are continuously evolving thereby increasing the need for current, relevant research studies.

WHY LEARN ABOUT RESEARCH METHODS?

Whether you choose a career in public health practice or are interested in working in other areas of public health, foundational knowledge in research methodology is essential for many reasons. First, it is important to understand how evidence is created. How do we know what intervention works best to increase vaccine uptake? How much physical activity do we need to decrease the risk of chronic disease? What policies are most effective in increasing access to healthy food? Evidence is needed to answer these questions, and it is research that builds the evidence.

In public health practice, two questions are foundational: (a) What are we trying to change? (b) What is the best way to achieve that change? *Evidence-based public health (EBPH)* is term used to describe decision-making for interventions on the basis of the best available scientific evidence by systematically using data and information, and considering community preferences. EBPH is modeled after evidence-based medicine (EBM), in which rigorous research informs best practices. However, the types of research studies performed in public health may differ from those contributing to medical evidence (i.e., randomized controlled trails [RCTs] may not be relevant for every public health issue). EBPH creates a higher likelihood of successful programs and policies being implemented and a more efficient use of resources.[10]

Evidence is gathered using the scientific method, which is the process of systematically observing and assessing to test hypotheses. A term often used in conjunction with the scientific method is *empirical research*. This refers to using data from systematic observations to inform conclusions. These observations can be quantitative, qualitative, or a combination of the two. **Quantitative methods** (discussed more in the section "Phases in the Research Process") use maximum objectivity and precision in order to produce generalizable findings. An example of a quantitative method would be a survey with multiple-choice response options. **Qualitative methods** (covered in the section "Categories of Research Purpose") are more flexible than quantitative methods, and these methods may evolve over time as the research progresses. Holding interviews and hosting focus groups are two examples of using qualitative methodology.

Empirical Research

Both forms of observations can be used in **mixed-methods** study design. In a mixed-methods study, the researcher combines both quantitative and qualitative methods in a way that best answers the research question or achieves the study aim. Using mixed-methods helps overcome inherent limitations by balancing the strengths and weaknesses of quantitative and qualitative methods. For example, a mixed-methods study would be useful if a researcher is interested in exploring poor dietary intake in a community. The researcher might want to investigate food access and choice; that is, what food is available and what influences food purchases? In order to get the information needed, a researcher might count the number of places to buy food and report the categories and prices of food available (quantitative). They might also interview a sample of local residents to gain their perspective on which stores they choose to buy food from and what influences this choice (qualitative). The combination of data from the interviews with the objective counts can provide more comprehensive information about food access in that community than either method alone. There are several different types of mixed-methods research, and these are defined in Table 1.2.

TABLE 1.2 FOUR TYPES OF MIXED-METHODS RESEARCH

Type	Definition	Example
Sequential explanatory	Quantitative data collected and analyzed first, then qualitative data are collected and analyzed	A quantitative online survey of school principals is done on the implementation of federal food requirements. Data from the survey are analyzed. There was a question on the survey asking respondents whether they would be willing to be interviewed about this topic. Interviews with a select group of principals are conducted, and data from these interviews are analyzed.
Sequential exploratory	Qualitative data collected and analyzed first, then quantitative data are collected and analyzed	Focus groups are conducted with low-income mothers of infants about barriers to postnatal care. Data are analyzed and results help inform a larger quantitative survey on this topic.
Concurrent triangulation	Collected at the same time and analyzed concurrently	A park audit is performed on counts of people and the activities they are doing. Qualitative observations are done of social interactions in the park setting. Both types of data are combined for a comprehensive story of park use.
Sequential transformative	Either collected first but data analyzed together	Interviews are done with healthcare providers of community clinics and patient outcome data are collected. Both sets of data are analyzed together to inform recommendations on improving chronic disease self-management.

Source: Adapted from Creswell JW. *Research Design: Qualitative, Quantitative, and Mixed Methods Approaches.* 2nd ed. Thousand Oaks, CA: Sage; 2003.[11]

A second reason for learning about research methods is to gain skills in assessing research quality. All evidence is not created equally or reported accurately. Some evidence has no merit at all. **Pseudoscience** or "fake science" is not based on the scientific method. Common characteristics of pseudoscience are extreme claims, overgeneralizations, and lack of sound research. Even studies conducted using good science still should be assessed for quality of evidence. For example, suppose you read an article describing an association between diagnoses of hypertension and having houseplants. Hypertension risk is a concern for you, but before you throw away all of your houseplants, you should consider the following:

- *Was research done in lab? On animals? With people?* Learn more about the research setting and participants to identify relevance and generalizability. Although animal science can be the basis of research translation, there may be caveats to its interpretability to humans.
- *Was there a large enough sample? How was the sample selected?* There are formulas for appropriate sample selection and size (see Chapter 5, Sampling), but you can assume that the bigger the sample, the better the generalizability (the extension of research findings from a sample population to the population at large) and lower chance of error. Results from a convenience sample of 10 people will not produce the depth of evidence needed to impact practice.
- *Where was the research conducted and who funded it?* Research conducted in academic settings or private organizations that follow rigorous scientific integrity regulations are more likely to produce legitimate research than studies conducted by organizations representing certain industry sectors, which may increase the chance for biased reporting. For example, a 2011 study found that children who eat sweets tend to weigh less than those who do not.[12] However, the National Confectioner's Association, a trade group representing candy manufacturers, sponsored this study.
- *Are conflicts reported?* Conflicts of interest represent circumstances in which professional judgments or actions regarding a primary interest, such as the responsibilities of a researcher, may be at risk of being influenced by a secondary interest, such as financial gain or career advancement.[13] Most reputable journals require authors to report any conflicts of interest that might bias their findings.
- *Where was the article published?* Top journals require rigorous peer review prior to publication. This means experts on the topic assess the submitted manuscript and make recommendations on whether or not the journal should publish it. However, there is a growing number of "predatory journals." These journals look legitimate when they advertise to researchers, but typically charge a high fee to publish articles and do not include peer reviews as part of their article selection process. A list of predatory journals can be found at predatoryjournals.com/journals.
- *How do headlines compare to actual study?* Popular press and social media are commonly used to disseminate research to the public, but journalists may not always interpret research results correctly. Flashy headlines will get the public's attention, but may not be substantiated. It is best practice to read the original study upon which the popular press or social media article was based and use that to judge the merit of the headline hype.

A headline for an article in the *Economic Times* was "Mental health alert! Eat more raw fruits and vegetables to feel better!"[14] At first glance, it seems there is evidence for improving mental health by consuming raw fruits and vegetables. Upon investigating the original research article published in *Frontiers in Psychology*, it was clear that the results should be interpreted with caution.[15] Self-reported intake of fruits and vegetables in a sample of 422 young adults in New Zealand was associated with *some measures* of self-reported mental health. The authors report their findings provided evidence that the consumption of raw fruits and vegetables has a stronger relationship with mental health than the consumption of cooked or canned (processed) fruits and vegetables. The authors also report study limitations such as correlation design (no causation can be assumed) and use of nonvalidated food-recall measures.

Some health claims promoted by the media are not backed by science or evidence. You may have heard that the recommended intake of water is eight 8-oz. glasses daily or that we all should be getting 10,000 steps in per day. Do some online searching to see whether you can find the evidence upon which these recommendations are based, but do not spend too much time on it. The evidence for these exact recommendations does not exist.

An understanding of research methods can facilitate public health advocacy. The first step in gaining community or stakeholder support for an issue is by increasing their awareness of that issue. Research provides evidence to share to gain that support. Suppose a community has an increase in bicycle commuter–car crashes. Residents may be more likely to support funding for bike-lane improvements or a change in speed limit when they learn the extent of the problem. With research skills, you could plan a study to collect data by surveying or interviewing cyclists, drivers, and transportation planners. As a researcher, you would also know the importance of finding existing information (e.g., crash data, geographic information, city planning policies) to support your case. The information gained might also expose disparities among those affected. In addition, a skilled public health researcher would be able to assess strategies implemented successfully in other places, which might be applicable to this community. Translating research to advocacy does not stop with gathering data. Presenting your information to different stakeholder groups in an appropriate and effective way is another highly useful research skill that helps advocacy. Whether advocacy efforts are a part of your job or used to support a topic you are passionate about, research skills come in handy.

Learning about research methods helps you become a better consumer of research information. As mentioned previously, the media may not always accurately portray research results. Every day there are headlines about what is good for you, what causes or prevents diseases, or what is effective in improving longevity. It is common for current reports to conflict with yesterday's headlines (Exhibit 1.1). Knowing about research can help you scrutinize what is reported, prompting informed conclusions about the merit and quality of the studies. You can also become a good interpreter of these studies for family and friends who may ask for your opinion of the latest health trend. Has someone ever said to you, *"They say that (fill in the blank) is bad for you so I am not eating/drinking/doing it anymore"*? With research skills, you will be able to find out who "they" are and investigate whether or not their claims are based on evidence.

PHASES IN THE RESEARCH PROCESS

Research is the result of a systematic process used to collect and analyze information so conclusions can be made and the research topic is better understood. The ways in which different disciplines use research vary, but all adhere to a similar research process based on

EXHIBIT 1.1 CONFLICTING RESULTS OF RESEARCH STUDIES ON FOOD AND CANCER

	Protects against cancer	Causes cancer
Wine	▲▲▲▲▲▲	▲▲▲
Tomatoes	▲▲▲▲▲▲▲▲	▲▲
Tea	▲▲▲▲▲▲▲	▲▲▲
Milk	▲▲▲▲▲▲	▲▲▲▲
Eggs	▲▲▲	▲▲▲▲▲
Corn	▲▲▲▲	▲▲▲▲▲
Coffee	▲▲▲▲	▲▲▲▲
Butter	▲▲	▲▲▲▲▲▲
Beef	▲▲	▲▲▲▲▲▲▲

▲ = One medical study

Source: Data from Schoenfeld JD, Ioannidis JP. Is everything we eat associated with cancer? A cookbook review. *Am J Clin Nutr.* 2013;87(1):127-134. doi:10.3945/ajcn.112.047142.[16]

the scientific method. There are six core phases in the research process. Each of the phases outlined in this section is also discussed in greater detail in subsequent chapters. This general overview helps frame the process from beginning to end, and lays the foundation for the rest of the book. It is important to note that although the phases are numbered and may seem sequential, sometimes the process is not linear. Unexpected changes or new revelations that occur during one step may require revisiting or modifying previous steps.

Replicability of research is vital in building an evidence base. If you carefully document your steps during the research process (as well as any adaptations), you will make it easier for other researchers to conduct comparable studies. As mentioned previously, a single study will not provide enough evidence for a definitive research conclusion. Additional research is needed to concur or refute existing findings so as to develop comprehensive, evidence-based best practices. Figure 1.1 shows the phases of research as a cyclical process in which one ends up back at the beginning: Research is the basis for more research.

Phase 1: Identify a Research Topic

In this phase, the researcher identifies an area of interest for which more knowledge is needed. Research ideas can be generated in many different ways. They can come from everyday

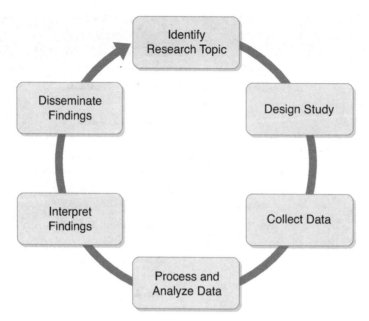

FIGURE 1.1 **Phases in the research process.**

observations, such as seeing people choose to take the escalator instead of the stairs. *What would it take to get people to choose the more active option?* Research ideas can also come from personal interest. If an elderly relative struggles to report her self-measured blood-pressure readings to her doctor because she struggles with the healthcare center's online program, a research question might be, *"What are the barriers to using online disease self-management programs for older adults?"* Sometimes common research topics (e.g., smoking) can be explored in different ways or with different subsets of the population to make them unique. This initial phase also includes reviewing the literature on the topic of interest and developing a conceptual framework on which to base your study. A conceptual framework is a methodological and analytical model, usually based on theory, that helps guide research projects. In quantitative studies this phase culminates with the development of a hypothesis.

Example: Your doctor's office just started a program in which they send you several text-message reminders about getting your flu shot. You find the messages serve as good reminders because you scheduled and received your shot. You are interested to know whether people who get the reminders are more likely to get flu shots than those who do not get the reminder texts. Upon searching the literature, you find there are many published studies and even several systematic reviews on this topic. However, you find very few of the studies included older adults who are Hispanic. You can narrow your study to this population focus to fill a research gap. The literature provides great ideas for the development of a conceptual framework. Finally, you hypothesize these interventions would be similarly effective in this population as in non-Hispanic older adults.

Phase 2: Design the Study

The most appropriate study design to choose is dependent on several factors. The feasibility of the study, in relation to sample population, budget, and time frame, should be considered. How easy will it be to access the population of interest? Will you have a large enough sample to support the design you choose? Are the costs of the study design consistent with your research budget? Budgeting and timeline planning for research is described in Chapter 8, Developing Budgets and Timelines for Research Studies, and are vital to study-design selection. The literature from Phase 1 can be a source of ideas for the best study-design fit. Several different designs may be appropriate for your research, with one exception. If determination of causation is required to answer your research question, then a randomized controlled trial (RCT) study design is needed. (More information about RCTs is found in Chapter 6, Quantitative Study Designs: Experimental). Data collection methods are also planned in this step. What type of information do you need? What is the most appropriate way to get this information from the population of interest? Will you use existing tools or create new ones? Cost is also a consideration when planning data collection. If your study involves human subjects, the level of participant burden in data collection may require monetary incentives. Incentives can be costly for larger samples.

Example: For the study on text-based flu-shot reminders, you find out that you can apply for access to de-identified health information from a healthcare center serving an older Hispanic community that just started a text-reminder program. The center is implementing this program in phases, and only patients whose last name begins with A to M got the reminders last flu season. Considering your budget and timeline, you decide on a quasi-experimental pre–post study with a comparison group. You will compare flu-shot uptake between patients with last names beginning with A to M to patients with last names beginning with N to Z the year prior to the text reminders as well as the year of the reminders. The data is already collected, and although it would be great to explore perception of this program through interviews, it is not feasible due to the de-identified nature of the data available.

Phase 3: Collect Data

During this phase you will use predetermined, systematic strategies to gather and measure information on variables of interest. Data collection differs in many ways depending on the approach used: quantitative, qualitative, or mixed method. No matter which approach you use, quality assurance and quality control are two important components of this phase. Quality-assurance strategies include planning and using a standard data-collection protocol. This facilitates consistency among the research team. Quality-control measures, such as data monitoring, can help identify errors during data collection. If a system of data monitoring is in place, issues with data collection can be resolved. For example, if data monitoring reveals no one is answering question 3 on your online survey, you can investigate and identify whether there is a faulty skip pattern or whether the question is not clear to participants. Changes can be made, saving data collection from a potential calamity. Documentation of the data collection protocol and the quality-control procedures you implemented is useful for dissemination (Phase 6 of the process). This information can be added to the methods section of academic papers and can be shared with others interested in replicating the study.

Example: In the flu-shot text-reminder study, the data is already collected through electronic health records (EHR). Because your agreement with the health center does not allow you to identify information, names and addresses are excluded. You request data for age, gender, race/ethnicity, employment status, marital status, health status, and vaccination record. You then find out the healthcare center is interested in people's perception of the reminder program and asks you to conduct focus groups. You go back to Phase 1 to look at the qualitative literature and plan for a mixed-methods study, and in round two of Phase 2, you develop your focus-group protocol. You implement two focus groups (in Spanish), one with people who received the texts and got their flu shots, and one with people who received the texts but did not get their flu shots.

Phase 4: Process and Analyze Data

After collection, the data needs to be prepared for analysis. The type of preparation varies by the method of data collection. If you used paper surveys, the data needs to be entered into a database or statistical software program. Data from online surveys can be imported to preferred databases easily. Preparation also includes identifying missing, out-of-range, or incomplete data. You will need to document and justify how you address these variable issues. Variables can be recoded into units that match the analytic methods used. Typically, quantitative data analysis goes from simple to complex, starting with descriptive characteristics. The type of analytic methods used depend on the research question or hypothesis.

Processing and analyzing data differs in qualitative research. Numbers are the unit of analysis in quantitative data; words are the focus of qualitative data. Qualitative data is typically recorded during collection (e.g., in focus groups) and transcribed into pages of verbatim text. Analysis depends on the theoretical basis being used. Typically, large amounts of text are grouped, condensed into themes, and summarized. This can be a done by hand or using a software analysis program intended for qualitative research.

Example: You receive the data from the EHRs and prepare for analysis. Because you are only interested in Hispanic older adults (age 65+), you use the race/ethnicity and age variables to pull out your sample for analysis. You then recode the variables into categories because that is needed for the type of analytical method you are using (e.g., yes/no for flu shot instead of date of shot). You compute descriptive statistics for all variables, and then conduct your comparative analysis of group outcomes. The focus group discussions were recorded and transcribed, and the text transcriptions uploaded to qualitative-analysis software. After reading through the text a few times, you and your team develop a codebook, and assign codes to all of the text. The codes are grouped together and you summarize the grouped codes into themes.

Phase 5: Interpret Findings

The next step after analyzing data and reviewing the results is interpretation. In this phase, the researcher describes the importance of the patterns and relationships that exist in the results. Reporting on the statistical significance (or lack of) is a big part of this phase in quantitative studies. It is important to discuss the extent to which analytic test results support or contradict the hypothesis developed in Phase 1. Not achieving a level of statistical significance is still a valid result that needs to be reported. Null findings help build the evidence base for public health recommendations as much as positive results. Only publishing positive findings in academic research (publication bias) can skew the overall knowledge on the topic, and negatively impact public health recommendations. Reporting limitations of the study is a necessary part of this phase. Many types of biases can affect results. Factors, such as sampling error, self-reporting, the weaknesses of the measures used, and limited generalizability, are limitations that are commonly reported.

Interpretation also includes comparison to other qualitative or quantitative studies. The researcher suggests reasons for similarities or differences among other results reported in the literature. Knowledge gaps and additional research questions may emerge from these comparisons. Research begets research.

Example: Your comparison of the text-message versus no-text-message group data reveals no difference in the percentage of older, Hispanic adults who get flu shots. In this study, text-message reminders did not impact the recipients. The patients who participated in the focus groups mentioned that they did not look at their mobile phones consistently. They used the phones more for talking than texting. This could be one reason for the null findings. A recurrent suggestion from the focus-group participants was to use phone calls instead of texts. Past literature reveals high effectiveness of text-message reminders in increasing flu-shot uptake for the general population. Your findings conflict with this. You reason that text reminders may be less effective in older adults, and add supporting evidence of differences in mobile phone use by age and race/ethnicity. You then add information from other text-message health interventions (blood-pressure management and weight loss), and report the concurring finding that these strategies are less effective for older adults.

Phase 6: Disseminate Findings

Sharing research findings with others is the final phase of the research process. The typical sequence used when reporting findings is background, methods, results, discussion, and conclusion. It is also helpful to summarize findings using a sentence or two to describe the implications of results for research and practice. In the past, dissemination only included publishing results in an academic journal for other researchers. We now know the importance of **audience segmentation**, in which dissemination strategies are tailored to specific groups. Important consumers of public health research information include practitioners, policy makers, advocacy groups, and the general public. The way in which research findings are presented should fit the needs of each of these groups. For example, policy makers are likely to prefer short summaries rather than lengthy research reports. Results should be given in plain language if the general population is the target audience. Methods of delivery of information also vary. Webinars, social media, and press releases are all ways in which researchers can share their work to a broad audience. It is important to know the preferred methods of acquiring information of the target audience in order to disseminate results effectively.

   Example: You decide to share your results with several different groups. First, you write a manuscript for submission to a reputable public health journal. Because the healthcare center was supportive of your work, you develop a PowerPoint presentation to be delivered to clinic staff. You also prepare a poster presentation for an upcoming public health conference on technology and health intervention and create a brief infographic to hang in the clinic waiting rooms.

CATEGORIES OF RESEARCH PURPOSE

Research studies vary in purpose. Some studies aim to explore new topics or take an initial step toward understanding a new or unfamiliar topic. The objective of other studies may be to rigorously evaluate a program or intervention. This variation is useful as it helps to build a more comprehensive evidence base for public health topics.

   The research purpose frames the study throughout the entire research process. For example, the research question and study design for an exploratory study on access to birth control for migrant workers would be very different from a study whose aim was to test an intervention to increase birth control access in this population. Data collection differs by research purpose, too. It is more acceptable to rely solely on qualitative data collection for exploratory studies than it is to use qualitative methods only in a rigorous evaluation.

   There are four generic ways to categorize the different purposes for public health research. These categories are often described in sequence, where specificity of the research increases with each level. The first and most flexible purpose for research is **exploration**. Exploratory studies aim to investigate something new or understudied. It can serve as preliminary research to other studies. Another category of research purpose is **description**. In descriptive studies, the researcher describes what is observed based on the tenets of the scientific method. These studies aim to answer "what" questions. The third category of research purpose is **explanation**. Explanatory studies go beyond just describing something. They aim to identify why things occur. In an explanatory study, the researcher will not just report differing rates of health disparity by zip code, but analyze why the rates differ. **Evaluation** studies may encompass the other three types of research purpose in order to identify the effectiveness of programs, policies, or interventions.

FINAL THOUGHTS ON THE IMPORTANCE OF RESEARCH IN PUBLIC HEALTH

Chances are you read or heard some headline related to health research today. Thinking about what led to the headlines is a good first step on your journey to understand research methods. After reading this chapter you should have a better understanding of why research is important to public health and what you can gain by learning about research methods. This chapter provides the foundation for the rest of the book, where components of the research process are discussed in detail.

CHAPTER DISCUSSION QUESTIONS

1. Why should training in public health include research methods?
2. Why might health research be misunderstood by the general public? What are some past examples of how information that was falsely presented affected health behaviors?
3. What aspects of public health research could contribute to health equity? What are some ways to encourage researchers to make sure their work addresses this?
4. What health headlines have you read recently? After reading this chapter, how would you go about investigating the merit of the study?

RESEARCH PROJECT CHECK-IN

What Interests You?

In a research methods course, students are often required to plan and conduct an actual research study as a form of applied learning. A research project starts with a topic of interest. After reading this chapter, you may have been thinking about a public health topic you would like to know more about. Or maybe you are interested in health issues related to a specific population. Sometimes the ideas are difficult to narrow down into a research topic that is interesting yet still feasible to conduct in a semester. Make a list of research ideas and rate each one by your level of interest, importance to public health, and practicality. Keep the top-ranked ideas for further exploration.

PUBLIC HEALTH RESEARCH METHODS IN REAL LIFE

All Public Health Publications Are Not Equal

Sonia was 6 months into her new job as project manager for a community center when she was thankful for her research methods training. The mission of the "Something To Do" center was to improve health and wellness of local children by providing structured activities, academic tutoring, and mentorship during after-school hours. The center was located in a small town of 20,000 residents about 60 miles outside of a large metropolitan area. Many residents had jobs working at the local fruit-processing plant and lived barely over the poverty line. Their shiftwork schedules at the plant were mostly inflexible. When school budget cuts eliminated the after-care programs in the two elementary schools in town, residents were left with few options for childcare.

At the beginning of the school year, a major television network publicized a news story about young children being left home alone because parents had no other choice. This publicity motivated a group of private donors to fund the community center to fill the gap left by the school budget cuts. The center had been operating for 2 years and showed positive impact on the lives of local children by providing them a safe and healthy place to spend their after-school hours.

The director of the center has a background in business and fund-raising. She is great at financial management and operations, and is well liked by the staff. Sonia was hired as the person to oversee programmatic initiatives at the center, especially related to health and wellness. She loves her job and is putting her public health training to good use. One day, Sonia was called into the director's office. She went to the meeting thinking some operational issue was the topic of concern. It turned out that one of the donors gave the director a newspaper article about a new intervention proven effective at helping children make healthy food choices. She wanted Sonia to read the article and investigate the program, and report back to the donor. The main component of the intervention was to provide unlimited processed, high-fat snacks to children so they eventually tire of them and make healthier choices. The article indicated that children in this intervention reduced their body mass index (BMI) and increased fruit and vegetable consumption.

Sonia remembered the criteria for assessing evidence that she learned in her research methods class. The article she was given came from an online news source called *NowUknow.com*. Sonia had never heard of this source. As she read the article, she determined that there was a lot of hype about the intervention without much evidence to back it up. The article did include a quote from a researcher who tested the intervention and a link to the original paper. The original paper did not come up when Sonia searched the literature databases most often used in public health. After some digging on the Internet, she finally found it. It was in a journal called *Affairs and Issues in Child Nutrition*. Sonia wrote many research papers on childhood nutrition during her master's program and had never heard of this journal. She then did what she was taught to do: Assess the study on which the claims were based. As she read the paper, she found that not only was the sample size composed of only 10 children, the study design was highly flawed. No pretest data were collected, there was no comparison group, and few valid statistical tests were run on the data. She also noticed the absence of any study limitations and author conflicts of interest. The Barkley Corporation was listed as the funder of the study. When she looked into the Barkley Corporation, she found it was the parent company of a multimillion-dollar snack-food manufacturer.

Sonia also noticed text in small print on the first page "Paper submitted 08/01/19. Paper accepted for publication 08/10/19." That only left 9 days for peer review—something her professors told her never happens—the process takes at least a few months! She recalled hearing about "predatory journals" and did an internet search. Sure enough, *Affairs and Issues in Child Nutrition* was listed as a journal in which authors pay large amounts of money to publish their work without going through a credible process of scrutiny for research rigor by peer review.

She typed up her notes and would NOT be recommending this intervention for children in the center. She found several other evidence-based and well-researched healthy-eating programs to suggest. She was very glad to have the research background and skills to be able to investigate health claims. If she did not know how to assess the validity of public health research, the children in her center might have been exposed to an ineffective intervention (not to mention too much junk food) and serious health consequences. In the end, her director thanked her, and given Sonia's information, the donor realized he should steer clear of suggesting programs he knew little about.

Critical Thinking Questions

1. Many people think that just because something is published, the research is valid. Have you ever encountered a situation like the one Sonia experienced? How did you convince anyone involved to reconsider their beliefs?
2. How can people who are not trained in public health learn about the importance of critiquing research?
3. Predatory journals are becoming a real challenge to legitimate peer-reviewed publications. What are some strategies or policies to limit or eliminate them?
4. One of the benefits of paying to publish articles (such as with legitimate open-access options) is that everyone can have access to your work, even if they do not subscribe to the journal or have access to the journal through a university. This is of benefit to practitioners, other stakeholders, and the public looking for evidence or information on public health topics. Predatory journals also provide free access to everyone. How do you feel about this open-access policy? Should everyone have access? Why or why not?

COUNCIL ON EDUCATION FOR PUBLIC HEALTH FOUNDATIONAL KNOWLEDGE AND COMPETENCIES

Foundational Knowledge

Profession and Science of Public Health

- Explain the role of quantitative and qualitative methods and sciences in describing and assessing a population's health.
- Explain the critical importance of evidence in advancing public health knowledge.

REFERENCES

1. Centers for Disease Control and Prevention. About chronic diseases. 2017. Accessed July 5, 2019. https://www.cdc.gov/chronicdisease/about/index.htm

2. United States Census Bureau. Older people projected to outnumber children for the first time in history. *Newsroom*. 2018. Accessed July 5, 2019. https://www.census.gov/newsroom/press-releases/2018/cb18-41-population-projections.html

3. United Health Foundation. American health rankings. 2018. Accessed July 5, 2019. https://www.americashealthrankings.org

4. Robert Wood Johnson Foundation. What is health equity? A definition and discussion guide—RWJF. 2018. Accessed July 5, 2019. https://www.rwjf.org/en/library/research/2017/05/what-is-health-equity-.html

5. Centers for Disease Control and Prevention. History of the surgeon general's report on smoking and health | CDC. 2017. Accessed July 5, 2019. https://www.cdc.gov/tobacco/data_statistics/sgr/history/index.htm

6. Centers for Disease Control and Prevention Office on Smoking and Health. Smoking and tobacco use. Electronic cigarettes. 2019. Accessed July 5, 2019. https://www.cdc.gov/tobacco/basic_information/e-cigarettes/index.htm

7. National Institue on Drug Abuse. Electronic cigarettes. 2019. Accessed July 5, 2019. https://www.drugabuse.gov/publications/drugfacts/vaping-devices-electronic-cigarettes

8. Henriksen A, Haugen Mikalsen M, Woldaregay AZ, et al. Using fitness trackers and smartwatches to measure physical activity in research: analysis of consumer wrist-worn wearables. *J Med Internet Res*. 2018;20(3):e110. doi:10.2196/jmir.9157

9. Sepah SC, Jiang L, Ellis RJ, et al. Engagement and outcomes in a digital diabetes prevention program: 3-year update. *BMJ Open Diabetes Res Care*. 2017;5(1):e000422. doi:10.1136/bmjdrc-2017-000422

10. Brownson R, Fielding J, Maylahn C. Evidence-based public health: a fundamental concept for public health practice. *Annu Rev Public Health*. 2009;30(1):175–201. doi:10.1146/annurev.pu.30.031709.100001

11. Creswell JW. *Research Design: Qualitative, Quantitative, and Mixed Methods Approaches*. 2nd ed. Thousand Oaks, CA: Sage; 2003.

12. O'Neil CE, Fulgoni VL III, Nicklas TA. Association of candy consumption with body weight measures, other health risk factors for cardiovascular disease, and diet quality in US children and adolescents: NHANES 1999–2004. *Food Nutr Res*. 2011;55(1):5794. doi:10.3402/fnr.v55i0.5794

13. Romain PL. Conflicts of interest in research: looking out for number one means keeping the primary interest front and center. *Curr Rev Musculoskelet Med*. 2015;8(2):122–127. doi:10.1007/s12178-015-9270-2

14. Mental health alert! Eat more of raw fruit and vegetables to feel better. *Econ Times*. n.d. Accessed July 5, 2019. https://economictimes.indiatimes.com/magazines/panache/mental-health-alert-eat-more-of-raw-fruit-and-vegetables-to-feel-better/printarticle/63816329.cms

15. Brookie KL, Best GI, Conner TS. Intake of raw fruits and vegetables is associated with better mental health than intake of processed fruits and vegetables. *Front Psychol*. 2018;9:487. doi:10.3389/fpsyg.2018.00487

16. Schoenfeld JD, Ioannidis JP. Is everything we eat associated with cancer? A cookbook review. *Am J Clin Nutr*. 2013;87(1):127–134. doi:10.3945/ajcn.112.047142

ADDITIONAL READINGS AND RESOURCES

Brownson RC, Baker EA, Deshpande AD, et al. *Evidence-Based Public Health*. 3rd ed. New York, NY: Oxford University Press; 2017.

Barbot O. Getting our heads out of the sand: using evidence to make system wide changes. *Am J Prev Med*. 2012;42(3):311–312. doi:10.1016/j.amepre.2011.11.007

Maher D, Ford N. A public health research agenda informed by guidelines in development. *Bull World Health Organ*. 2017;95:795–795A. doi:10.2471/BLT.17.200709

Medical Research Council, Chief Scientist Office, and University of Glasgow. Understanding health research: a tool for making sense of health studies. 2019. https://www.understanding-healthresearch.org/notice/1

U.S. Department of Health and Human Services, National Heart, Lung and Blood Institute. Study quality assessment tools. 2019. https://www.nhlbi.nih.gov/health-topics/study-quality-assessment-tools

Literature Search and Research-Question Development

*Research is to see what everybody else has seen and to think
what nobody else has thought.*
> —Albert Szent-Gyorgyi, Hungarian scientist

INTRODUCTION

A fundamental task in developing a research study is to review the existing literature. A **literature review** is a summary and synthesis of published information on a subject area. The main goals of the literature review are to familiarize yourself with what is already known about the topic and to identify gaps that justify your study.

Because of the volumes of published studies and the time-consuming nature of this step, undertaking a literature review can daunt even the most seasoned researcher. Today's researchers should be thankful for technological advancements, which make a literature review tremendously easier than it once was. Just a few decades ago, a literature search meant trips to the library to sift through printed and bound volumes of academic journals. If the library did not have a specific journal needed, you would request it from the librarian and wait for it to arrive via mail—not email. Luckily, technology has evolved to make searching and accessing many types of articles, books, and reports easier. Online databases, search engines, and accessible electronic copies of research publications improve the ease of this important step in the research process.

WHY REVIEW THE LITERATURE?

The information uncovered during the literature review contributes to every phase of the research process. In the earliest phases of topic identification, a review of published studies may give insight into new ways of looking at your research topic. What exists in the literature also implicitly identifies what *does not* exist among studies on your topic. This is called a **research gap**. Suppose your topic of interest is healthy food policies in schools. You find many studies on policies covering school cafeteria food, but no studies on policies for food served at school sporting events. From searching the literature, you identified a gap and can narrow your research focus. Maybe you found many studies on food policies in urban school districts, but none representing rural districts. Specificity of a research topic in terms of setting or population characteristics can also help narrow and clarify your research purpose. Table 2.1 shows ways a broad public health research interest can be made more precise.

Published research provides details on many important aspects of a study that are helpful in planning research studies. As discussed in Chapter 1, The Importance of Research in Public Health, replication of studies builds the evidence base. Academic research articles include detailed descriptions of study methodology so the study can be reproduced, and

TABLE 2.1 IDEAS FOR NARROWING RESEARCH FOCUS		
Broad Topics	**Characteristics of Population**	**Characteristics of Setting**
Obesity	Age	Urban/rural
Vaccinations	Race/ethnicity	Community
Healthy eating	Gender	School
Physical activity	Education	Policy jurisdiction
Preventive screenings	Social support	Healthcare
Depression/anxiety	General health status	Places of worship
Healthy aging	Mobility	Childcare settings
Access to healthcare	Geographic location	Government agencies
Policies affecting health		
Environmental health		
Infectious disease		
Sexual health		
Health education		

results compared across studies. A literature review may help identify the most relevant methods of data collection on a specific topic or with a unique population. No researcher wants to waste time creating something that already exists. The literature provides a gateway into existing tools for measuring public health issues. Currently, many journals with online access allow authors to supplement their publication with appendices, such as surveys or other data-collection tools used. A researcher can also request the tool from the author, if it is not readily accessible.

The literature is valuable when planning data-analysis methods. There are myriad choices in statistical tests and ways to analyze data. Assessing how other researchers computed analyses could help inform your decisions about the best ways to analyze data for the topic of interest. All journals list contact information for at least the correspondence author of the article. If you need more information on analysis than what is provided in the publication, you can contac the author with your questions.

In addition, the Discussion section of scholarly publications usually includes any limitations of the study and ways in which it could have been improved. The "lessons learned" from researchers who have completed their studies are like a bequest to the research community. Researchers designing new studies can proactively address limitations reported from past studies. For instance, a literature search results in several articles on family-based interventions to reduce sugar-sweetened-beverage consumption in children. Intervention effectiveness varies by type of intervention and setting, but nearly all of the discussions include a limitation of "longer follow-up needed." Researchers should incorporate this suggestion when planning for new intervention study designs on this topic.

Literature-review information is highly relevant to the interpretation phase of the research process. In this phase, you contextualize your study findings in relation to past studies. The literature provides a foundation for determining how your research fits within the existing knowledge. In the interpretation phase, you compare and contrast your results with past studies, and hypothesize why differences might exist. You can also use the literature review to demonstrate how your study filled a research gap and contributed to existing information on the topic.

LITERATURE-REVIEW NOMENCLATURE

A basic literature review is the simplest form of gathering and summarizing research information and is the method most likely used by beginning researchers. However, there are other types of reviews that warrant mention. You may come across publications of these specialized reviews when you do your own search.

Systematic reviews: A systematic review involves collecting and analyzing all evidence that answers a specific question. This includes a comprehensive and exhaustive search of the literature and critical analysis (not just a summary like in a basic review) of the search results. The goal of a systematic review is to provide an evidence-based answer to a very specific research question.[1] Cochrane, an organization formed to facilitate the creation of evidence-based health choices, developed the standard protocol for systematic reviews. This organization also houses an online, searchable database for published systematic reviews (www.cochranelibrary.com/cdsr/reviews).[2] Another guide for systematic reviews is Preferred Reporting Items for Systematic Reviews and Meta-Analyses (PRISMA). PRISMA provides an evidence-based minimum set of items for reporting in reviews (www.prisma-statement.org).

A good example of how systematic reviews are used in public health is the *Guide to Community Preventive Services*; referred to as the *Community Guide*. The *Community Guide* uses systematic reviews of effectiveness and economic evidence to determine whether an intervention approach works and is cost-effective. See Exhibit 2.1 for an example of the *Community Guide* recommendations, or visit the interactive website (www.thecommunityguide.org).

Meta-Analysis: A meta-analysis combines the quantitative results of a number of different studies into one report to create a single, more precise, and robust estimate of effect.[3] Data from individual studies are combined to reach new statistical conclusions. These conclusions are statistically stronger than the individual studies because combining results also increases the number and diversity of the study population. Figure 2.1 shows an example of how results from a meta-analysis are presented.

Scoping Review: A scoping review is a preliminary assessment of potential size and *scope* of available data. These reviews are most suited for a body of literature that is complex

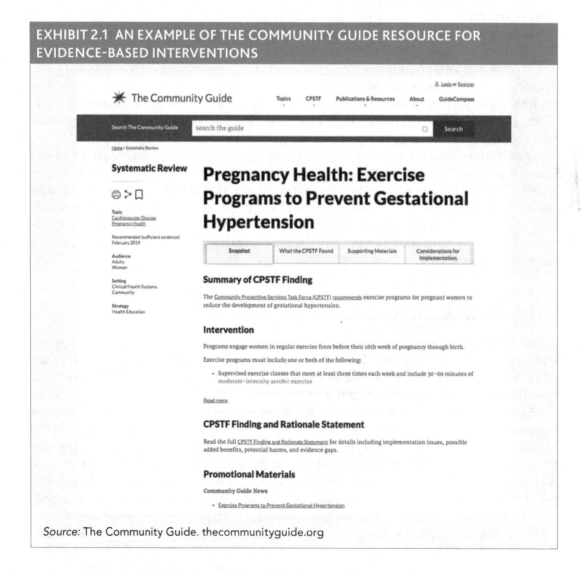

EXHIBIT 2.1 AN EXAMPLE OF THE COMMUNITY GUIDE RESOURCE FOR EVIDENCE-BASED INTERVENTIONS

Source: The Community Guide. thecommunityguide.org

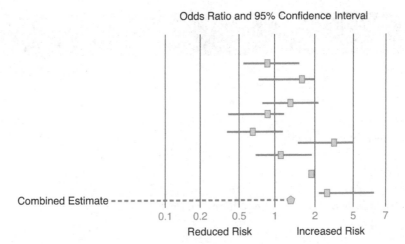

FIGURE 2.1 **Example of presentation of results from a meta-analysis.**

or heterogeneous and that would not be well suited for a systematic review.[4] Scoping reviews are useful for assessing emerging evidence when it is still unclear what other, more specific research questions can be posed.[5] Scoping reviews can be conducted prior to a systematic review.

Review-of-Reviews: There is a good chance many systematic reviews are published on well-researched topics. For example, a quick database search to find studies using "smoking and systematic review" as search terms yields almost 3,000 results. Instead of synthesizing individual studies, this type of review combines relevant data from systematic reviews and meta-analyses to inform recommendations within a specific topic.

Scholarly research publications in academic journals are the most widely accepted resources for literature reviews in public health. Because journals vary in quality, researchers look to a quality-rating score called the **journal impact factor.** The impact factor is the average yearly number of citations of recent research from that journal within the past 2 years.[6] Although impact factor is not a perfect measure of quality, it identifies the top journals in each field. Researchers would not continually cite studies if they had no merit. Examples of public health journals and impact factors are listed in Table 2.2. Another measure of journal quality is its presence in the Medline or PubMed databases. The National Library of Medicine rigorously reviews journals for critical elements of quality prior to index approval. Newer journals might lack an impact factor or index not because of poor quality, but because they have not been around long enough to fully determine their value. To make sure the journal source is legitimate, be sure to check the list of predatory journals mentioned in Chapter 1, The Importance of Research in Public Health.

Other resources can supplement your literature review of academic research articles. **Grey literature** is a term that describes documents produced for purposes other than commercial publication (i.e., academic journals). Examples include conference abstracts, government reports, or industry documents. One reason searching grey literature is important is because it is one way to address **publication bias.** Studies with positive, significant results are more likely to be published in academic journals compared with those having negative or no results. Including some grey literature may balance this bias within your research topic.

TABLE 2.2 EXAMPLES OF PUBLIC HEALTH JOURNALS RANKED BY IMPACT FACTOR, 2018	
Journal Title	Impact Factor
The Lancet Public Health	11.6
Annual Review in Public Health	9.49
Tobacco Control	6.22
International Journal of Behavioral Nutrition and Physical Activity	5.55
American Journal of Preventive Medicine	4.43
American Journal of Public Health	4.38
Social Science & Medicine	1.72
Journal of Adolescent Health	3.97
Preventive Medicine	3.45
European Journal of Public Health	3.07
International Journal of Public Health	2.73
BMC Public Health	2.56
Journal of Urban Health	2.15
Public Health Reports	2.04
Australian and New Zealand Journal of Public Health	1.91
Maternal and Child Health Journal	1.74
Journal of Immigrant and Migrant Health	1.58
Journal of Community Health	1.52
Asian Pacific Journal of Public Health	1.39
Journal of Public Health Management and Practice	1.37
Canadian Journal of Public Health	1.25

Before you start your search, consult your librarian. Librarians are superheroes when it comes to doing literature searches. They can demonstrate how to access and use your school's online databases and guide you on the most efficient ways to search your topic of interest. Their assistance will save you time and frustration.

CONDUCTING A LITERATURE REVIEW

There are several basic steps to follow when conducting a literature review. Much like the phases in the research process, sometimes the literature-review steps may not be sequential. You might have to go back to previous steps to modify things before progressing. Do not underestimate how much time this task can take. Even though database searching has come a long way since the "old-fashioned" visits to the library, a good literature review takes time. Also, keep track of your search methodology during each step. Record search terms, modifiers, number of results, number eliminated and the reason for exclusion, and so on. This is important information to add to the methodology section of your research report. The basic procedure for reviewing the literature is as follows:

1. **Get a general overview of the topic.** Public health issues are broad and complex. If you have trouble selecting a specific research problem, your first step would be to scan some articles to get a sense of what some options might be. You might identify ways to narrow your focus after reading a few articles. Let's say you are interested in studying diabetes. There are many different ways to frame research within this topic: Type 1 or type 2 diabetes? Prevention or maintenance of this condition? All ages or a specific age group? Any specific race/ethnicity? Or maybe you want to research a specific disease outcome such as renal failure. Once you have identified the specific concepts, you can proceed to step 2.
2. **Select search terms.** Using the key concepts developed in step 1, list all the different versions of the words and related terms. It is helpful to create a table with a column for each concept. See Table 2.3 for an example. Look up terms in a thesaurus to get ideas to add to your comprehensive list. You can also scan some titles of related papers and see what words other researchers use to frame the topic. The methodology reported in published systematic reviews can also help populate your search-term list. Authors typically describe in detail the words they used in their searches. If the review is related to your key concepts, their search terms might be relevant for your work.
3. **Select appropriate databases.** Most journals are indexed in one or more electronic databases. These databases can be accessed through university libraries, and even some public libraries. Common databases used for public health research are listed in Table 2.4. All of the main databases include academic journals, but the additional content may vary. Some encompass book chapters, dissertations, and even popular sources. Make sure you know the type of literature needed for your search. Most databases allow selection of resource types (e.g., journals only). It is best to use more than one of the databases to ensure a comprehensive search. Through a university library database, you will have access to many full-text documents. Your librarian can help you with any interlibrary loans needed for full-text articles in journals to which the school may not subscribe. It may be tempting to just use an Internet search engine to find resources for

TABLE 2.3 EXAMPLE OF DEVELOPING KEY CONCEPTS INTO SEARCH TERMS

Key Concepts: What is the relationship between healthy food access and obesity in women?

obese	food	access	woman
obesity	groceries	accessible	women
	grocery	accessibility	female
	fruit		
	fruits		
	vegetable		
	vegetables		

your literature, but you may not get quality results. You may also have to sort through a large number of results, many of which will not be relevant to your key concepts. Google Scholar (scholar.google.com) is better than a general Internet search, but is not as precise as other literature databases and may not link to all available full-text documents.

4. **Apply search strategies.** There are several steps you can take to make your search results more relevant and easier to manage. The first is to use *Boolean operators* (AND, OR, and NOT) to narrow or broaden your search. AND narrows the results through inclusion (e.g., women AND depression). OR broadens the results (e.g., depression OR anxiety). NOT narrows your topic through exclusion (e.g., depression NOT postpartum). Some databases use AND NOT, so be sure to check the database guide. *Truncation* is a way to find all words that come from the same stem word. Databases differ in the truncation symbols used, but are typically * $!. For example, SCHOOL* finds school, schools, schooled, schooling, and so on. You can also include whole phrases in your searches by putting the phrase in quotation marks (e.g., "Every Student Succeeds Act"). Limiting your search to academic journals, English language, and publication years helps increase the precision of your results. Make sure to use publication-year limits relevant for your research topic. If you are conducting an historical view, older articles are necessary. If you are researching concepts that have shifted or developed over time, more current literature is more appropriate (e.g., online or app-based interventions). There is no standard recommendation for how "current" research is defined. Many researchers aim for articles published within the last 10 to 15 years, unless a paper represents a landmark study.

5. **Review your results.** Sorting through search results is the next step. Look at the results and decide whether they meet your needs. If you have too many resources, consider applying more limits. If you have too few results, broaden your search by finding more synonyms or adding broader terms. No matter how well you develop your search strategy, there will be some resources not relevant to your research. You can eliminate articles as you review titles and abstracts. There may even be a second

TABLE 2.4 COMMON LITERATURE DATABASES USED FOR PUBLIC HEALTH RESEARCH	
Database	Description
PubMed www.ncbi.nlm.nih.gov/pubmed/	A free search service of the National Library of Medicine, which provides citations in life sciences and biomedical topics dating back to 1966. This database contains more than 30-million citations and abstracts of peer-reviewed literature. PubMed Central is included in PubMed and contains full-text articles resulting from federally funded research.
CINAHL/EBSCO www.ebscohost.com/nursing/products/cinahl-databases/cinahl-complete	The CINAHL database includes broad content such as nursing specialties, speech and language pathology, nutrition, and general health. It includes searchable cited references for more than 1,500 journals.
ERIC ies.ed.gov/ncee/projects/eric.asp	The ERIC provides access to journal and nonjournal (grey) literature from 1966 to present. This database includes over 1,000 journals and 1.6 million indexed items.
Academic Search Complete/EBSCO www.ebsco.com/products/research-databases/academic-search-complete	A searchable indexing service covering social science, education, psychology, and other subjects. Contains journals, magazines, newspapers, and other media. Coverage includes more than 10,000 journals and reports, as well as conference proceedings and other sources.
PsychINFO www.apa.org/pubs/databases/psycinfo/	Contains abstracts and index records of nearly 2,500 psychologically relevant, archival, scholarly, peer-reviewed journals, books, and dissertations. This database contains over 4.7 million records.

CINAHL, Cumulative Index to Nursing and Allied Health Literature; ERIC, Education Resources Information Center.

round of elimination after reading the full-text papers. Select the articles for review and create a way to summarize the text. One way to do this is to create a summary table. Identify the important components of the articles in the table as you read them. An example of a literature review summary table is shown in Table 2.5. Condensing the text of articles into summaries organized and presented in one place makes it easier to synthesize the material in the next step. If you realize you need more information after reading and summarizing selected articles, there are shortcuts to finding more information without doing an entire search. Academic researchers tend to have an area of expertise. Try searching for articles by author name to find other relevant resources. You can also look at the references within articles you already

TABLE 2.5 EXAMPLE OF A LITERATURE REVIEW SUMMARY TABLE

Citation	RQ/Study Aims	Study Design and Sample	Analysis	Main Results	Limitations	Other Notes
Eyler et al.[7]	Gain insights into high school athletic directors through key informant interviews about sports participation fee policy implementation in a sample of U.S. school districts	Qualitative Interviews 12 athletic directors	Qualitative, constant comparative coding with some a priori developed codes	Terms used by ADs differed. Main reasons for fees differed. All had waivers for students who could not pay the fee. Most felt fees were not affecting participation, but opposition remained	Sample limited to a few states. Limited by qualitative method, not generalizable. Did not compare to actual policy.	Study results are to inform future study. Equity angle is interesting. Low-income more affected?

ADs, athletic directors

reviewed for additional information. Some databases have a "similar articles" sidebar, highlighting publications that might be of interest based on your initial search. Proceed to the outline step if you reviewed a sufficient amount of information to serve as the basis of your research.

6. **Outline and write your review.** A basic literature review is similar to the Background or Introduction section of a research article. You recently read a lot of these in the previous step, so you should have a good sense of how to present your research information. It's a good idea to start with an outline. Outlining a review structure before you write the full text makes the process less daunting and more organized. Your review should begin with an introduction to the topic. What is it? Why is it relevant to public health? Who does it affect? The first paragraph often contains statistics (e.g., prevalence) about the issue to give the reader a sense of the extent of the issue. Start with a broad scope of the topic and then narrow the focus. Next, describe how the topic has been studied. The key to a good review is not just reporting about each study one after another, but to compare and contrast the research. Describe how this topic has been studied and synthesize results. Be sure to critique the studies on the basis of their limitations. Discuss the samples used. Who was studied? Who is missing? Was diversity or disparity addressed? After a thorough discussion of the studies, report on any gaps related to your topic and justify the importance of addressing them. Conclude with your research question or study objective.

QUESTIONS TO CONSIDER WHEN READING ARTICLES

- What were the research aims?
- How was the aim achieved?
- What were the limitations of the study?
- What are the lessons learned from the study?
- What might you do differently?
- What do authors recommend for future study?
- How could you build on this work?

DEVELOPING RESEARCH QUESTIONS

You might have started your literature review with a specific research question in mind. However, the process of searching and summarizing information on the topic may have given you new insight or reasons to modify your original question. The question can evolve as a result of a research review. A good research question provides structure for the rest of the research process.

There are several issues to consider when developing a research question. First, the research purpose can affect how you write your question. If you were conducting an exploratory study your question would be very different from one used in an evaluation study. It is also important your research question is not too broad. For example, "Why do children get disciplined in schools?" is too broad. Narrowing the focus to "What are the main causes of disciplinary action in middle school children in the St. Louis Public School District?"

would hone in on a precise research interest. A precise research question sets boundaries to help maintain a manageable study. In the discipline example, the setting and population are clearly stated. The concept of "disciplinary action" can be defined and measured. Develop measurable research questions. Make sure what you propose in your research question is feasible, especially if there is a short time frame available to you, such as a 15-week semester. Other aspects of feasibility include ethical considerations, budget, and partners or stakeholders needed for the study. See Table 2.6 for examples of research questions.

TABLE 2.6 EXAMPLES OF RESEARCH QUESTIONS

Too Narrow	More Broad
What is the vaccine uptake rate in Anytown, United States?	How does the education level of parents impact vaccine uptake rates in Anytown, United States?
This can be answered with a simple statistic. Questions that can be answered with "yes/no" should be avoided.	This shows specificity. The results will provide opportunities for discourse.
Too Broad	**More Focused**
What are the effects of childhood obesity in the United States?	How does childhood obesity correlate with bullying in elementary school children?
This questions is very broad and beyond the scope of one research paper.	This question has a very clear focus to facilitate progression through the steps of the research process.
Too Simple	**More Complex**
How are workplaces addressing employee mental health?	How does company size affect the extent to which it addresses employee mental health?
This can be answered simply with a search and so may not be suitable for analysis.	This adds another component to the study, allowing results to be compared and contrasted.
Too Objective	**More Subjective**
How much water do preschool-aged children consume?	What is the relationship between water consumption and children's weight?
This will result in merely a number without the need to collect data beyond factual assessment.	This will likely lead to comprehensive data that can be analyzed to form an argument.

Reviewing the literature can be an ongoing process. Whether you are working on a project over a long period of time or stick to the same topic of research throughout your career, you need to stay current on published research. New articles come out daily. One way to keep current is to use Internet research alerts. You can sign up online to receive regular updates on published literature for your needs. Check which alert services are available for your topics of interest.

REFERENCES

Evidence is built on the accumulation of research. When you write your literature review, you will no doubt refer to the work of others. Documenting where you obtained your information is required. This shows the reader which concepts and facts are your own, and which originated from other sources. Referencing the work of others gives credit to past researchers and adds credibility to your own work. Citing other sources signifies to the reader that you are informed about the topic and have used past research to cultivate your perspective. Another reason accurate referencing is needed is that it can lead the reader to the original resource used in case they want to learn more. In addition, citations are a metric for assessing the quality of journals and contribute to the accumulated scholarship of the academic researcher.

Researchers (and students of research methods) must correctly identify the sources of information or are at risk of **plagiarism**. *Plagiarism* refers to using the work of another without crediting the original source. Plagiarism is a form of cheating that can result in negative consequences. Your school or university will likely have an academic integrity policy outlining plagiarism. Be sure to read it before starting your literature review. Librarians are a good source of information about how to avoid plagiarism.

There are some guidelines as to when to cite a source. The general rule is that you must acknowledge a source if you mention something that is not your original idea. You need to cite the source any time you summarize, paraphrase, or use direct quotes. Data, facts, and images also require citations. The only exemption for this general rule is that you do not have to cite any information considered **common knowledge**, or information most people know (e.g., George Washington was the first president of the United States). The concept of common knowledge is a bit vague. If you are in doubt as to whether or not something needs to be cited, err on the side of caution and cite it.

The preferred ways in which you acknowledge the work of others within your document vary by discipline. The reference styles require the same information be given for the original source, but the information is presented differently within the text and the bibliography. Psychology and many other social sciences adhere to the style of the American Psychological Association or APA reference style. In this style, the author and publication year are included in parentheses after the statement. Although there is no standard reference style for public health as a discipline, many public health researchers use the style of the American Medical Association (AMA) for citations and bibliography. In AMA style, sequential superscript numbers are used for in-text citations. The *American Journal of Public Health,* for example, adheres to AMA style. Style guides for each format are available online or through your library.

TABLE 2.7 COMPARISON OF CITATION SOFTWARE PROGRAMS[A]

	EndNote[b]	Mendeley[c]	Refworks[d]	Zotero[e]
Cost[f]	●		●	
Desktop	●	●	●	●
Web-linked	●	●	●	●
Easiest to learn		●		●
Many output styles	●	●	●	●
Export to other programs	●	●	●	●
Write and cite	●	●	●	●
Easy to manage large libraries	●		●	
Share with others	●	●	●	●

Notes: [a]There are other programs available. Do a search for citation-management software to learn about programs not listed in this table. [b]endnote.com. [c]www.mendeley.com. [d]www.refworks.com/refworks2. [e]www.zotero.org. [f]Your school or university might have a subscription to EndNote or Refworks. You may be able to access these for free. EndNote Web Basic with 2 gigabytes of storage is free, but desktop software has a fee.

Citation Software

One of the greatest technological advancements in helping researchers report their work is citation software. Incorporating citation software in your work will save you a tremendous amount of time. Instead of inserting each reference by hand, and manually developing the bibliography, citation software programs allow you to create references directly from databases or the Internet. These programs also allow you to choose and change the reference style easily. If you develop your literature review in APA style, but then your instructor requires AMA, you can quickly make this change without retyping everything. Another feature of these programs is their ability to create online reference databases, which can be shared with others. This is helpful for group projects or research teams. Your school or university may subscribe to a specific program and support the program with trainings or technical assistance. See Table 2.7 for a comparison of popular citation software. Please note that even though the programs do much of the formatting work for you, they are not foolproof. You still need to check the citations and bibliography for accuracy.

CHAPTER DISCUSSION QUESTIONS

1. How would the *process of* a literature review on gender representation in smoking advertisements differ from a review of rural access to telehealth?
2. Describe reasons for searching both scholarly research and the popular press for a research study investigating fad diets.
3. What are the pros and cons of refining your research question before your literature review compared with after your literature review?
4. How is the literature review applicable to other steps in the research process?

RESEARCH PROJECT CHECK-IN

What Does the Literature Tell You?

By now, you should have narrowed your research interest somewhat. You can limit your topic even more with information from the literature (public health and other disciplines). Conduct a review of the literature to take note of past studies on the topic. You can learn a great deal from results, but also look to the literature for lessons learned and ideas for future studies. As you read more information on your topic, you will begin to refine the research idea into a specific research question or study aim. These statements will guide you during the rest of the research process.

PUBLIC HEALTH RESEARCH METHODS IN REAL LIFE

The Search Is On

Samar has been asked to summarize the literature on the topic of sexually transmitted diseases and older adults in order to identify a research gap, which can then be turned into a compelling grant application. Thinking there may not be that much information published, he starts with a simple search in Google Scholar by typing "Older Adults and Sexually Transmitted Diseases." To his surprise, the search results in over 300,000 documents. It will take him a long time to even read all the titles. Samar remembers from his research methods class that there is an art and science to conducting literature searches. He refers back to his course notes and creates a plan.

The grant's call for proposals mentions the spike in sexually transmitted disease prevalence in older adults after the widespread use of sexual performance-enhancing drugs. Samar does some further online investigation and finds the first drug for erectile dysfunction was approved by the U.S. Food and Drug Administration in 1998. His first strategy to narrow his literature search is to limit the time period. He decided to search back 10 years after the first drug was introduced. He selects a range of 2008 to the current year. Still in Google Scholar, his search results in 19,000 articles. This is too many to review in time for the grant application deadline.

Remembering how the university librarians helped him with his literature searches when he was in his public health program, he decided to go back to his notes and try their strategies. First, he made a table to help identify the key concepts with synonyms and related phrases. He tried to think of all the ways "older adults" and "sexually transmitted diseases" might be identified in the literature. Because it was important that articles contained both of these topics, he came up with several search strategies using Boolean operators, such as AND, OR, and NOT, so he could link the concepts of older adults and sexually transmitted diseases. He also generated a list of different word endings so he could use common truncating and stemming symbols if needed. He remembered his librarian's advice and abandoned Google Scholar to access a more comprehensive and searchable literature database through his library.

He ran two variations of the search and still generated a list of too many papers to review. He tried limiting the search to only papers (not books or book chapters) in English and from the United States. The list remained too long. Then he had an idea about a strategy he used for one of his research projects in school. He decided to search only for review papers on the topics. The review papers would give him summaries of past research and enough information about what is already known about this topic. Finally! There were 27 review articles published about older adults and sexually transmitted diseases. Upon further inspection of the results, he omitted three duplicates and four that were not relevant. This left him with 20 papers to review so as to come up with research-gap recommendations.

As he read the papers, he paid particular attention to the Discussion sections. Most of the authors compared and contrasted the results from the papers reviewed and made recommendations for future research. He also made notes on the populations represented in the papers reviewed. One factor he noted was that in spite of national recommendations for sexually transmitted disease testing for healthcare providers, not much has been reported about the healthcare provider's perceptions of implementing these guidelines with their patients. No paper reported findings by race/ethnicity of the provider or the patients. He found the gap. Samar summarized the literature and recommended a grant proposal to explore the perceptions of sexually transmitted disease testing for older adults among diverse healthcare providers. His public health literature searching skills came in handy for what could have been a monumental task. He was confident that he completed a comprehensive search and proud of his summary and recommendation.

Critical Thinking Questions

1. What other ways could Samar have come up with a topic for the grant proposal?
2. How would the results have changed if the time limits were different? What if the search only included articles from the last 5 years?
3. What other ways could Samar have limited his search? What populations or parameters could he have used?
4. How might looking into the popular press help find articles on this topic? Do you think this would have been a good strategy? Why or why not?
5. Abstracts usually offer great summaries, but sometimes articles you gather may not be relevant. How might a high number of nonrelevant articles be a challenge to the literature review?
6. The topic of healthcare providers and implementation of sexually transmitted disease testing on older adults is still quite broad. How else might this be narrowed in focus?
7. Describe how you would use the findings of this literature review to shape an intervention.

COUNCIL ON EDUCATION FOR PUBLIC HEALTH FOUNDATIONAL KNOWLEDGE AND COMPETENCIES

Foundational Knowledge
Profession and Science of Public Health
- Explain the critical importance of evidence in advancing public health knowledge.

Foundational Competencies
Evidence-Based Approaches to Public Health
- Interpret results of data analysis for public health research, policy, or practice.

REFERENCES

1. Centers for Disease Control and Prevention. Systematic reviews. 2015. Accessed July 8, 2019. https://www.cdc.gov/library/researchguides/systematicreviews.html

2. Cochrane Organization. What is Cochrane? 2019. Accessed July 9, 2019. https://www.cochrane.org/news/what-cochrane

3. Tatsioni A, Ioannidis JPA. Meta-analysis. In: Quah SR, ed. *International Encyclopedia of Public Health*. 1st ed. Elsevier; 2008:117–124.

4. Daudt HM, van Mossel C, Scott SJ. Enhancing the scoping study methodology: A large, interprofessional team's experience with Arksey and O'Malley's framework. *BMC Med Res Methodol.* 2013;13:48. doi:10.1186/1471-2288-13-48

5. Arksey H, O'Malley L. Scoping studies: towards a methodological framework. *Int J Soc Res Methodol.* 2005;8(1):19–32. doi:10.1080/1364557032000119616

6. Munn Z, Peters MDJ, Stern C, et al. Systematic review or scoping review? Guidance for authors when choosing between a systematic or scoping review approach. *BMC Med Res Methodol.* 2018;18(1):143. doi:10.1186/s12874-018-0611-x

7. Clarivate Analytics. Impact factor. 2019. Accessed July 9, 2019. https://clarivate.com/essays/impact-factor

8. Eyler A, Valko C, Serrano N. Perspectives on high school "pay to play" sports fee policies: a qualitative study. *Transl J Am Coll Sports Med.* 2018;3(19):152–157.

ADDITIONAL READINGS AND RESOURCES

American Medical Association. AMA Manual of Style. 2019. Accessed July 9, 2019. https://www.ama-manualofstyle.com

Centers for Disease Control and Prevention. Systematic reviews. 2015. Accessed July 9, 2019. https://www.cdc.gov/library/researchguides/systematicreviews.html

Community Preventive Services Taskforce. The Community Guide: our methodology. 2018. Accessed July 9, 2019. https://www.thecommunityguide.org/about/our-methodology

Iskander JK, Wolicki SB, Leeb RT, et al. Successful scientific writing and publishing: a step-by-step approach. *Prev Chronic Dis.* 2018;15:180085. doi:10.5888/pcd15.180085

Paultasso M. Ten simple rules for writing a literature review. *PLoS Comput Biol.* 2013;9(7):e1003149. doi:10.1371/journal.pcbi.1003149

Ethics in Public Health Research

Nihil de nobis sine nobis.
          —"Nothing about us without us," Latin motto

INTRODUCTION

Research in both medicine and public health has contributed to significant societal benefits. Research, however, has ethical implications. Ethics can be defined as the doctrine of conduct applicable to individuals or organizations. Within a research context, these principles relate to the conduct of the researcher. The public health researcher has a moral and professional obligation to search for knowledge in a way that is explicit, transparent, and truthful.

Public health ethics evolved from medical ethical principles. Bioethics or clinical ethics are based on the principle of doing what is best for the *individual* patient by balancing benefits and risks. Public health has a societal responsibility to protect and promote *population* heath. There is a community context embedded in the ethical principles of public health research that goes beyond consideration of the individual patient. There is a need to balance the rights and needs of the community with the benefits and costs of the research to that community.

According to the U.S. Department of Health and Human Services (DHHS), **human subjects research** is research involving "a living individual about whom an investigator conducting research obtains (a) data through intervention or interaction with the individual or (b) identifiable private information."[1] Human subjects research also includes the use of previously collected biological specimens (e.g., tissue, blood) if those samples are linked to identifiers. Interactions between researchers and participants could refer to communication or other interpersonal contact. This definition covers different types of data, from blood and tissue samples to survey information. If you gather information from people in any way, it likely involves human subjects research. Even if you do not collect the data yourself, it can still be considered human subjects research if the data has information that identifies the original research participants.

HISTORICAL CASES SHAPING RESEARCH ETHICS

Protection of human subjects is based on a history of unethical research transgressions. Decades ago, there was little concern for people who participated in research studies. The emphasis was on the scientific outcome rather than protecting those whose bodies were used to provide information. The Nazi experiments during World War II are an example of horrific and unethical medical experimentation. German physicians conducted medical experiments on concentration camp prisoners without their consent and with dire consequences. In 1946, an American military tribunal proceeding resulted in criminal prosecution of 23 of these German physicians for their willing participation in war crimes and crimes against humanity.[2] This prosecution led to the development of the Nuremberg Code in 1948, which was the first international document to promote the protection of human subjects in research.[2]

Although a milestone in the history of research ethics, the development of the Nuremberg Code was not an end to unethical practices with human subjects. In 1932, the U.S. Public Health Service began a 6-month study to document the progression of syphilis. Partnering with the Tuskegee Institute, the research goal of the "Tuskegee Study of Untreated Syphilis in the Negro Male" was to track the natural history of syphilis in African American men in order to justify treatment programs for this population. The study initially involved 600 African American men (399 with syphilis and 201 without the disease) from Macon County, Alabama.[3] The study participants were told the purpose of the study was to treat "bad blood"; a term investigators thought equated to local understanding of syphilis. Men enrolled in the study received free medical exams, free meals, and money for burial. Those enrolled did not receive proper treatment to cure their illness. Rather than ending the study after the initial 6 months, the study continued for 40 years.[4]

In 1972, the Associated Press published a story about the Tuskegee study. As a result of this story, the Assistant Secretary for Health and Scientific Affairs appointed an ad hoc advisory panel to review the study. This panel found the men in the Tuskegee study were misled by researchers and not informed of the actual purpose of the research. The panel also confirmed the men were not given adequate treatment for their disease, even after the efficacy of using penicillin to treat syphilis became standard medical practice. The study was deemed "ethically unjustified" as the risks to the subjects outweighed the benefit of the knowledge gained, and was ceased.[3]

As more information became public, the demand for reparations for the unjust treatment of Tuskegee-study participants emerged. In 1973, a class-action lawsuit was filed on behalf of study participants and their families.[3] In 1974, lifetime medical benefits and burial for participants were included in a $10 million settlement, and expanded in 1975 to include wives, widows, and offspring. In 1997, President Bill Clinton issued a formal apology and declared government responsibility for the failure to protect participants and the unethical practices within the Tuskegee syphilis study.[4]

A more recent example of unethical public health research is the Havasupai "Diabetes Project." The Havasupai Tribe is a federally recognized Indian Tribe residing in the Grand Canyon of northwestern Arizona.[5] In 1989, Arizona State University (ASU) researcher John Martin partnered with Havasupai tribal members to investigate the epidemic of diabetes mellitus, which was having a devastating effect on the health and well-being of the tribe. The goals of this partnership were to provide education on nutrition and physiology, facilitate testing for diabetes or diabetes risk, and to make genetic testing available to identify potential genetic correlates of the disease among tribal members.[6,7] Professor Martin sought the help of human genetics professor Theresa Markow to assist with the genetic testing for the diabetes project. Professor Markow saw an opportunity to tie in her own research interests (schizophrenia) to the Havasuapi project. She applied for and received a grant to study schizophrenia among Havasupai members without tribal permission.

This was the first project to obtain permission for collecting blood samples, as blood holds significant cultural and spiritual worth to the tribe. Researchers stressed to the Havasupai Tribal Council that diabetes was the sole outcome of interest, yet the written consent form to have blood drawn indicated the purpose of the research was "to study the causes of behavioral/medical disorders."[6,7] After studying the samples, Markow concluded diabetes was not related to genetics due to the lack of genetic variation among tribal members. Markow continued using the samples along with an unauthorized review of tribe members' medical charts to study schizophrenia.

In 2003, Professor Martin invited a tribal member who was also an ASU undergraduate student to a dissertation defense on population migration theories related to the Havasupai blood samples. When the presentation began, the student realized the misuse of the blood samples of her tribe. Migration studies conflict with the cultural beliefs on tribal origins. In addition, the doctoral student defending the dissertation did not have tribal permission to use the samples for his study. After the Havasupai Tribal Council was informed of the research misconduct, the tribe issued a Banishment Order.[8]

BANISHMENT ORDER

"The Havasupai Tribe has recently been informed by reliable sources that Havasupai blood collected by ASU has been distributed to others for research, and that research may have been conducted on Havasupai blood, by ASU and by others, for purposes unrelated to diabetes or any other medical disorder, all in violation of the consent given by Havasupai members. ASU, its professors and employees are, from this date forward banished from the Havasupai Reservation."[9]

ASU, Arizona State University.

Investigation into the Havasupai study revealed most of the published academic papers, articles, and dissertations referencing Havasupai blood were not related to diabetes.[6] The Havasupai tribe filed two separate lawsuits against ASU Board of Regents, and these cases lasted nearly 6 years before resolution. The main issues of concern were lack of informed consent, violation of civil rights through mishandling of blood samples, unapproved use of data, and violation of medical confidentiality.[8] The outcome of the lawsuit included several required actions, including returning the remaining blood samples and documentation materials to the tribe members. Researchers also were mandated to provide a list of anyone or any place that received the samples and to cease all IRB approval of research using the blood samples.[8]

The Tuskegee and Havasupai studies are two examples of unethical research. These studies took advantage of vulnerable populations and the lack of informed consent violated the right of the participants. In the Havasupai case, the researchers blatantly disregarded cultural priorities over scientific inquiry. These studies highlight the need for guidance and oversight in research to ensure ethical implementation.

ETHICAL GUIDANCE FOR PUBLIC HEALTH RESEARCH

Better guidance for ethical research is often the outcome of unethical research. The prosecution of German physicians who conducted the Nazi experiments resulted in the Nuremberg Code. The Tuskegee syphilis study lawsuit resulted in specifications for informed consent and better governmental oversight. The outcome of the Havasupai "Diabetes Project" trial was increased awareness of the importance of cultural competence in research. Although there is no guarantee oversight and guidance will safeguard against all future ethical issues in public health research, several documents have evolved to outline best practices.

International Guidance

NUREMBERG CODE (1948)

As indicated previously, the Nuremberg Code was a direct result of prosecution of those who conducted the Nazi experiments. It was the first international document to emphasize human rights among research participants. The Nuremberg Code outlines 10 principles that remain requirements for current ethical research practice. These include voluntary consent, ability to withdraw from the study, and the importance of research quality standards. See Exhibit 3.1 for the Nuremberg Code. Even though it is not an enforceable law, it is considered one of the most important influences in the history of research ethics.

DECLARATION OF HELSINKI (1964)

Building on the foundation of the Nuremberg Code, the World Medical Association developed the Declaration of Helsinki—Ethical Principles for Medical Research Involving Human Subjects.[11] Its primary audience is physicians, but components of the declaration have become standard for ethical conduct in all research with human subjects. The World Medical Association made several updates to the original 1964 document in order to adapt to advancements in science and technology. The current ethical principles not only cover human

EXHIBIT 3.1 THE NUREMBERG CODE

THE NUREMBERG CODE

1. The voluntary consent of the human subject is absolutely essential. This means that the person involved should have legal capacity to give consent; should be so situated as to be able to exercise free power of choice, without the intervention of any element of force, fraud, deceit, duress, over-reaching, or other ulterior form of constraint or coercion; and should have sufficient knowledge and comprehension of the elements of the subject matter involved, as to enable him to make an understanding and enlightened decision. This latter element requires that, before the acceptance of an affirmative decision by the experimental subject, there should be made known to him the nature, duration, and purpose of the experiment; the method and means by which it is to be conducted; all inconveniences and hazards reasonably to be expected; and the effects upon his health or person, which may possibly come from his participation in the experiment.

   The duty and responsibility for ascertaining the quality of the consent rests upon each individual who initiates, directs, or engages in the experiment. It is a personal duty and responsibility, which may not be delegated to another with impunity.

2. The experiment should be such as to yield fruitful results for the good of society, unprocurable by other methods or means of study, and not random and unnecessary in nature.

3. The experiment should be so designed and based on the results of animal experimentation and a knowledge of the natural history of the disease or other problem under study, that the anticipated results will justify the performance of the experiment.

4. The experiment should be so conducted as to avoid all unnecessary physical and mental suffering and injury.

5. No experiment should be conducted, where there is an a priori reason to believe that death or disabling injury will occur; except, perhaps, in those experiments where the experimental physicians also serve as subjects.

6. The degree of risk to be taken should never exceed that determined by the humanitarian importance of the problem to be solved by the experiment.

7. Proper preparations should be made and adequate facilities provided to protect the experimental subject against even remote possibilities of injury, disability, or death.

8. The experiment should be conducted only by scientifically qualified persons. The highest degree of skill and care should be required through all stages of the experiment of those who conduct or engage in the experiment.

9. During the course of the experiment, the human subject should be at liberty to bring the experiment to an end, if he has reached the physical or mental state, where continuation of the experiment seemed to him to be impossible.

10. During the course of the experiment, the scientist in charge must be prepared to terminate the experiment at any stage, if he has probable cause to believe, in the exercise of the good faith, superior skill, and careful judgment required of him, that a continuation of the experiment is likely to result in injury, disability, or death to the experimental subject.

Source: United States Library of Congress. *Trials of War Criminals before the Nuremberg Military Tribunals under Control Council Law No. 10.* Vol. 2. Washington, DC: U.S. Government Printing Office; 1949:181–182.[10]

subjects research, but also research on identifiable human material and data. See most the most current declaration (www.wma.net/policies-post/wma-declaration-of-helsinki-ethical-principles-for-medical-research-involving-human-subjects).

United States Guidance

BELMONT REPORT (1979)

The publicity of the Tuskegee Syphilis Study created the demand for government action to support ethical research. As a result, the **National Research Act** was signed into law in 1974. This Act created the National Commission for the Protection of Human Subjects of Biomedical and Behavioral Research. This commission was in charge of developing basic ethical principles for biomedical and behavioral research involving human subjects. In addition to the guidelines, the commission was tasked with developing a system of assurance that the research is conducted with the established ethical principles. In 1976, the Commission published the Belmont Report.[12]

The Belmont Report outlines ethical principles and guidelines for research involving human subjects. The three basic ethical principles of the Belmont Report are:

1. *Respect for Persons.* This principle encompasses three important facets of human subjects research. First, people involved in a research study should be capable of understanding the study activities and consequences of participation, and be able to make an informed decision about participation. Second, persons with diminished autonomy who might not be able to understand what they are being asked to do in a study, or who have limited capacity for free choice, are considered vulnerable populations and require additional protection. Respect for persons also covers the right to privacy. Incorporating strategies to protect privacy of study participants (e.g., identifiable data) is necessary.
2. *Beneficence.* Beneficence refers to first, doing no harm to human subjects; and second, maximizing the possible benefits while minimizing the potential harms. Harm can come in many different ways (e.g., physical, psychological, social) and must be considered broadly in an assessment of risks and benefits. For example, there may be a risk of injury in a physical-activity intervention. Anxiety as a result of trying to meet the demands of disease-management intervention is an example of psychological risk. Quitting smoking as a result of a tobacco-cessation program while your partner or friends remain smokers poses social risk. **Minimal risk** is defined by federal regulations as the probability and magnitude of physical or psychological harm from participating in research is no greater than that normally encountered in the daily lives, or in the routine physical or psychological examinations, of healthy persons.[1] In addition, considering the risk to the population at large is an important aspect of ethical public health research. It is vital to consider the benefit of the research to society as a whole while also calculating the risks of society if the research is not conducted. Risk can range from minimal to significant.
3. *Justice.* This term relates to the fairness of who should receive the benefits of the research and who should bear its burdens.[12] The benefits and risks should be distributed justly and equitably. There are several common ways in which people should be treated equally. Widely accepted formulations of just ways to distribute burdens and benefits include to each person (a) an equal share, (b) according to individual need, (c) according

to individual effort, (d) according to social contribution, and (e) according to merit.[12] There must be equity in sampling and participant selection if risks and burdens are to be fairly distributed. Selecting certain populations to participate in research because the studies may be high risk and other populations for low risk is an injustice. Systematically selecting certain populations (e.g., rural, poor) because of their specific life circumstances or perceived manipulability goes against the principle of justice. Justice in the research context also means that study subjects should be treated fairly, and this treatment should not be biased by cultural, racial, sexual, or other characteristics.

COMMON RULE (1991, RECENT UPDATES 2019)

The current safeguards to protect human subjects in research were significantly informed by the Belmont Report, and continue to evolve. In 1991, many federal agencies and offices (including the DHHS) adopted "The Federal Policy for Protection of Human Subjects," or the **Common Rule**. This rule applies to human subjects research conducted or supported by the agencies adopting it. Each institution that conducts research under the Common Rule is required to adhere to **Federalwide Assurance (FWA).** The FWA is written, legally binding assurance that the organization will comply with the Common Rule. The main requirements under the Common Rule include

- assuring compliance by research institutions;
- obtaining and documenting informed consent; and
- IRB membership, function, operations, review of research, and record keeping.

The Common Rule also outlines additional elements for protection of vulnerable populations in research. These include pregnant women, human in vitro fertilization and fetuses, prisoners, and children. Although the Common Rule specifies certain vulnerable categories, these guidelines were not intended to be exclusive, leaving the interpretation of vulnerability broad and open.

As research and technology evolve, the requirements for ethical human subjects research change. In January 2019, the federal office for Human Research Protections updated the Common Rule. One of the main changes to the 2019 version of the Common Rule was the revision of the definition of *human subjects*. The new definition was expanded to explicitly state inclusion of *identifiable* bio-specimens and specifications of consent for future research on these specimens. The updated definition states a human subject is

> A living individual about whom an investigator, whether professional or student conducting research: 1) obtains information or bio-specimens through intervention or interaction with the individual, and uses, studies, or analyzes the information or bio-specimens or 2) obtains, uses, studies, analyzes, or generates identifiable private information or identifiable bio-specimens.[1]

The 2019 updates also include a requirement for use of consent forms to provide potential research subjects with clear information about the study so they can make a more fully informed decision about participation. The consent forms for certain federally funded clinical trials are required to be posted on a public website. There are also new requirements to manage human subjects research compliance for multi-institutional studies. One of the updates to the Common Rule relevant to many public health research studies is the change in the way regulations apply to low-risk studies. There are now new categories for studies that are exempt from certain aspects of human subjects research protection requirements based on the low level of risk the studies pose to participants. This reduces the regulatory burden for the researcher, and allows more institutional attention to higher risk studies. The updated Common Rule can be found in the Electronic Code of Federal Regulations, Part 46-Protection of Human Subjects (www.ecfr.gov/cgi-bin/retrieveECFR?gp=&SID=83cd09e1c0f5c6937cd9d7513160fc3f&pitd=20180719&n=pt45.1.46&r=PART&ty=HTML).

INSTITUTIONAL REVIEW BOARDS (IRB)

As part of the Common Rule, any public or private entity, department, or agency receiving federal research funds is required to have an IRB.[1] The IRB provides regulatory and ethical oversight of research studies conducted within an institution. These boards function to ensure the protection of human subjects and ensure compliance with federal requirements. An IRB has the authority to review, approve, require modification, deny, or monitor all research activities under its jurisdiction. Exhibit 3.2 outlines IRB functions. Regulatory requirements on IRB membership exist to ensure objective and fair review of research studies. An IRB must include at least

- five members of varying backgrounds, both sexes, and more than one profession;
- one scientific member, one nonscientific member, and one unaffiliated member; and
- one member knowledgeable about regularly researched vulnerable groups.

Not all studies are equal in the level of IRB oversight needed. The levels of review are based on the potential risk to the participants in the study. For example, the risk to participants who complete an anonymous survey about neighborhood food access is low, compared with a study in which participants adhere to a specific nutrition intervention and provide blood samples to measure cholesterol. When preparing to submit a research project for IRB approval, most institutions have a process for determining the level of review needed through a series of questions about the study, population, and perceived risk. See Exhibit 3.3 for levels of IRB review.

EXHIBIT 3.2 FUNCTIONS OF AN INSTITUTIONAL REVIEW BOARD AS STATED IN U.S. FEDERAL POLICY FOR PROTECTION OF HUMAN SUBJECTS RESEARCH

An IRB should determine whether
- risks are minimized;
- risks are reasonable in relation to anticipated benefits, if any, and the importance of the expected knowledge;
- subject selection is equitable and attention is paid to vulnerable populations;
- informed consent will be sought and documented;
- there are adequate provisions for monitoring;
- adequate provisions to protect confidentiality; and
- additional safeguards for subjects vulnerable to coercion or undue influence.

IRB, institutional review board.

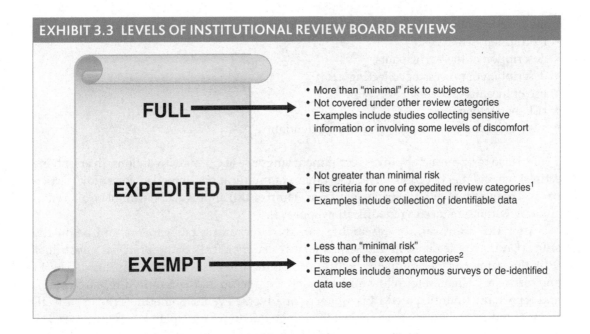

EXHIBIT 3.3 LEVELS OF INSTITUTIONAL REVIEW BOARD REVIEWS

FULL
- More than "minimal" risk to subjects
- Not covered under other review categories
- Examples include studies collecting sensitive information or involving some levels of discomfort

EXPEDITED
- Not greater than minimal risk
- Fits criteria for one of expedited review categories[1]
- Examples include collection of identifiable data

EXEMPT
- Less than "minimal risk"
- Fits one of the exempt categories[2]
- Examples include anonymous surveys or de-identified data use

In addition to federal IRB regulations, states or institutions may add their own additional provisions. The 10th Amendment to the U.S. Constitution transferred many powers of the federal government to states.[13] This creates inconsistencies between federal and state law in many cases, such as the regulatory landscape of marijuana use. Legalization of marijuana by some states has led to explicit distinctions on research involving this drug, since use and possession of this drug remains illegal in the majority of states. The U.S. Food and Drug Administration outlines strict guidelines and regulations for marijuana research with human subjects. Some institutions within states where possession and use of marijuana is legal (e.g., Oregon State University) added specific language to their research policies explicitly stating that studies on possession, use, or distribution of marijuana are prohibited unless the study complies with federal guidelines.[14]

The Institutional Review Board Review

Most institutions rely on an online process for researchers to use to provide study information for review. Typically, there are different requirements for behavioral versus biomedical research. Researchers need to be familiar with what is required in order to adequately prepare the information prior to filling out the IRB application. You must provide background information of the topic and reasons for the study. Other information that is needed for IRB applications may include

- sources of support (e.g., grant or other funding);
- study team members, their affiliation, and role in the project; (Note: All team members are required to have undergone Collaborative Institutional Training Initiative [CITI] training. See Exhibit 3.4 for more information.)
- whether or not the study is a clinical trial required to be in a federal registry;

- the study population, inclusion and exclusion criteria with justification;
- recruitment strategies;
- description of the participants;
- description of process of collecting data;
- use of incentives;
- risk management;
- strategies for ensuring privacy and confidentiality.

IRB also reviews and approves recruitment language (e.g., email invitations, flyers, phone scripts), your data-collection tools, and other communications intended for study participants. These documents are given an official stamp of IRB approval and cannot be altered in any way without requesting modification approval.

After IRB approval, the researcher can start recruiting participants and begin the study. Under the leadership of the primary researcher (called the *principal investigator [PI]*), the study can be conducted within the boundaries of what was approved. The PI and team are obligated to follow ethical practices, document the required research steps, and report any unanticipated consequences or adverse events. Sometimes the most well-thought-out research plans are subject to change due to unanticipated consequences. For example, if your research involves interviewing people who attend a community wellness center and that center has an infrastructure problem resulting in closure during the time of the study, you will have to modify your recruitment and inclusion criteria. *Adverse events* refer to unfavorable physical or psychological occurrence as a result of participation in the study. Suppose your study goal is to assess physical activity of employees in an average workday. To collect study data, accelerometers are secured to the upper arms of participants with an elastic band. If a participant has an allergic reaction to latex in the armband and has to drop out of the study, the PI is responsible for reporting this adverse event to the IRB. Institutional human subjects research offices can provide clarity on the extent to which unintended problems or adverse events should be reported during your study.

EXHIBIT 3.4 COLLABORATIVE INSTITUTIONAL TRAINING INITIATIVE

CITI was developed in 2000 as training course for human subjects research protections in medical research. The mission of CITI is to promote the public's trust in research by providing high-quality, peer-reviewed, web-based educational courses in research ethics. It was expanded in 2004 to include content for social and behavioral researchers. The training is designed to enhance the knowledge and professionalism of investigators, staff, and students conducting research in the United States and internationally. Most institutions require completion of the CITI courses prior to becoming involved in research involving human subjects, and offer access to certification for students. If you are interested in conducting public health research as part of your studies or in your career, completing the CITI training is recommended. For more information refer to your institution's Research Office or visit the CITI website (about.citiprogram.org/en/homepage).

CITI, Collaborative Institutional Training Initiative.

RESEARCH MISCONDUCT

According to the DHHS ORI, *research misconduct* means fabrication, falsification, plagiarism in proposing, performing, reviewing research, or in reporting research results. Violating federal or institutional regulations governing research can result in various levels of consequence. ORI works with institutions on misconduct investigations. Penalties of research misconduct include receiving a letter of reprimand, suspension or termination of the research project, imposing required research supervision, or banning the researcher from all federally funded grant activities. Research misconduct may have a detrimental effect on the public's health and safety. For instance, in spite of official retraction of Andrew Wakefield's famed study linking vaccines to autism, people still shun vaccines based on his false findings.

DHHS, U.S. Department of Health and Human Services; ORI, Office of Research Integrity.

Source: US Department of Health and Human Services, The Office of Research Integrity. What is research misconduct? Frequently Asked Questions. Accessed August 1, 2019. https://ori.hhs.gov/content/frequently-asked-questions#5.

INFORMED CONSENT

The need for informed consent is deeply rooted in the history of public health research. A major ethical issue in both the Tuskegee Syphilis Study and the Havasupai "Diabetes Project" was the lack of participant's consent to be involved in the research activities. Today, there are very specific requirements for the informed-consent process. Potential research participants need to be provided with clear and understandable information on which to judge their willingness to participate. Requirements for this information include what their involvement entails, the benefits and risks, the extent of confidentiality, and any compensation (incentives) they will receive. Potential participants must also be given information on the opportunity to choose not to participate or the ability to withdraw from the study without negative consequences. In addition, consent documents must include names and contact information of the principal investigator (PI) of the study and representatives of the institutional human research protection office. See Exhibit 3.5 for an example of an informed-consent document.

The consent process differs by research risk. For studies with greater than minimal risk, participants and a research team member must sign the consent document. These signed, unaltered documents need to remain on file for 7 years or the time period defined by the institution. An IRB may waive the requirement for a signed informed consent form if the study is deemed to have minimal risk, the potential harm from loss of confidentiality is low, or if the potential participants are from a cultural group or community in which signing forms is not the norm.[15] For some studies of minimal risk, an interview participant may consent over the telephone after being given the required consent information. Consent for participation in an anonymous online survey can be acquired by providing project information at the beginning of the survey and giving participants the choice to click options to either consent and participate in the survey or refuse participation.

A legally authorized representative can provide consent for research participants who may not be capable to provide consent. For example, a parent or legal guardian can provide consent for children in a research study. A child may also be able to **assent** to participate.

EXHIBIT 3.5 EXAMPLE OF AN INFORMED CONSENT DOCUMENT FOR AN ANONYMOUS ONLINE SURVEY

> FOR IRB USE ONLY
>
> IRB ID# 201616169
> APPROVAL DATE; 01/20/2018
> RELEASED DATE; 01/20/2018
> EXPIRATION DATE: N/A

As part of the Brown in Balance Wellness Initiative, we invite you to participate in a health survey. The purpose of this survey is to gather information on the health habits and risks in the Brown School community so we can plan the most effective wellness programs in the upcoming year. We will also use the information for baseline measures to help is set wellness goals.

If you agree to participate, we would like you to fill out this brief online survey. You may skip any questions you prefer not to answer. The survey will take approximately 10 minutes.

As an incentive for participating, you will have the chance to be entered into a drawing for one of four $25.00 bookstore gift cards. When you complete the survey, you will have the opportunity to link a database to enter your name and email for the drawing. Your name and email will not be connected in any way to survey information. You may skip the name and email link if you refuse the incentive.

We will not collect your name or any identifying information in the survey and it will not be possible to link you to your responses on the survey.

Taking part in this survey is voluntary. If you do not wish to participate, you can choose not to click on the survey link. You can also exit the survey at any time.

If you have any questions about the survey or the wellness initiative, please contact the project's lead researcher, Dr. Amy Eyler, at (314) 935-0129 or aeyler@wustl.edu. If you have questions about the rights of research participants, please contact the Human Research Protection Office, 660 S. Euclid Ave., Campus Box 8089, Washington University in St. Louis, St. Louis, MO 63110, (314) 633-7400, or (800)-438-0445, or email hrpo@wusm.wustl.edu.

Assent means a child's affirmative agreement to be involved in the research study. At the federal level, anyone over the age of 18 is considered an adult and can provide consent. However, states have different laws about age of adulthood. A child aged 16 may be able to legally sign a consent form and participate without a parent or legal guardian's approval. Some public health research with children can use parents' **"passive consent,"** or the researcher's assumption that a parent is permitting a child to participate. For example, researchers collecting data through surveys at school can send research study information home with students with an opportunity for parents to "opt out" and refuse their child's participation. These consent options must be carefully considered for relevance to the study and approved by IRB.[15]

OTHER ETHICAL CONSIDERATIONS

The concepts of privacy and confidentiality are integral to public health research ethics. **Privacy** refers to control over sharing information with others. The characteristics (i.e., cultural norms) of the study population may inform the level of privacy needed, as the importance of privacy may differ within groups. The greater the sensitivity of information collected, the greater the need for privacy in both data collection and management. People may be reluctant to share personal information in a group setting or in places where they may be overheard warranting private data collection. **Confidentiality** means information linking participants to their data (identifiers) will be kept private and not be available to anyone outside of the research study team. Names, addresses, or other identifiers assessed should be replaced with separate study identification numbers. The process of keeping data confidential must be outlined in order to obtain IRB approval. An IRB review will determine the level of safeguards needed to maintain privacy and confidentiality. Some public health research uses protected health information (PHI). The Health Insurance Portability and Accountability Act (HIPAA) of 1996 mandates provisions to protect the confidentiality of personally identifiable information obtained through healthcare. This law requires disclosure and authorization of the use of PHI.[16]

Anonymous data collection is common in public health research. **Anonymous** means there is no way to connect response data to the individuals providing that data. In anonymous research, the data does not include any identifiable information. Anonymity in data collection may increase response rate and decrease socially desirable responses. However, anonymity can be challenging in some research circumstances. Suppose you are collecting data from teachers in a small school district. The teachers fill out a survey, but do not provide names. They do report demographic characteristics such as gender and age. If the population includes certain demographic outliers (e.g., only one male, 36 years old), then that data is identifiable. In this case, the provisions for confidentiality risks should be outlined in the informed-consent document, as anonymity cannot be fully achieved.

IS DECEPTION IN RESEARCH ETHICAL?

Deception occurs when investigators provide false or incomplete information to mislead research participants. Beginning in 1961, psychologist Stanley Milgram conducted one of the most famous studies using deception. The purpose of the study was to explore obedience in taking orders from superiors. Participants (called "the teachers") were told to increase the level of electric shock given to participants (called "the learners") as punishment for incorrect responses to a word-recall question. The intensity of the shock increased with the number of incorrect responses. The learners were in another room, and the teachers were made to believe they were actually shocking the learners—but they were not. The majority of teachers obeyed orders to shock the learners to the highest level. After several iterations of the experiment, Milgram (1974) wrote *Obedience to Authority: An Experimental View* concluding that adults respond obediently when instructed by an authority figure even when inflicting harm on others.[30] This study had several ethical implications, including the use of deception, which Milgram argued was necessary in order to achieve truth.

Deception remains a research strategy, but its use in public health is quite different from that which was used in the Milgram studies. A review article by McCambridge et al. describes the use of deception in public health intervention trials on alcohol use in college students. Information on the study purpose was intentionally withheld from the study participants in order to achieve study aims in all three trials reviewed. The effect of knowing the true purpose of the study was a variable being studied in and of itself.[17] Today, the use of deception as a research strategy requires detailed justification to the IRB on why it is necessary for the study. A researcher using deception must also indicate whether this strategy might affect willingness to participate, increase risks to participants, and how participants will be debriefed after the study.

IRB, institutional review board.

The use of incentives in research can also pose ethical issues. **Incentives** are used to recruit or encourage people to volunteer to participate in research studies and compensate them for bearing the burden of participation requirements. Incentives can be financial (e.g., money, gift cards), services (e.g., transportation to data collection, medical tests, memberships), or products (e.g., fitness trackers, promotional items). There is a gap of knowledge on how to calculate fair amounts of compensation for time and effort of study participation. The ethical appropriateness of research incentives, especially financial, has been disputed. There is a concern that some monetary incentives increase the potential for coercion to participate.[18] Larger cash amounts for studies with higher than minimal risk are of most concern, and need careful IRB review. Another ethical issue is reporting or tracking of monetary incentives given to participants. Institutions often have a maximum allowable amount for cash or gift-card incentives due to required compliance with Internal Revenue Service laws. Because of this, they may require collection of participant Social Security numbers upon incentive distribution. Participants may be reluctant to provide this personal information and refuse study enrollment. This has the potential to bias the study's sample population. There is also an ethical concern related to timing of the incentive. The informed-consent document should clearly state when the incentive will be given to participants and to what extent they need to complete study requirements in order to be eligible to receive it.

BIAS AND CULTURAL CONSIDERATIONS IN RESEARCH

Diversity in public health research is necessary for reducing disparities and improving equity in public health practice. Researchers must possess proficient cultural competency skills in order to address this important issue. **Cultural competence** is defined as the ability to respect and respond to the cultural and linguistic needs of others.[19] This concept is relevant to healthcare, public health programs and services, and research. Awareness of the need for cultural competence increased with publication of the *Secretary's Task Force Report on Black and Minority Health (Heckler Report)* in 1985. This was the first federal documentation of health disparities in ethnic and racial minorities. Other federal guidelines were developed to help advance heath equity. In 1999, the National Institutes of Health developed the *NIH Strategic Research Plan to Reduce and Ultimately Eliminate Health Disparities* to identify gaps and set priorities related to addressing health disparities.[20] This plan was updated in 1994 and makes inclusion in the NIH-funded research a requirement by law.

> It is the policy of NIH that women and members of minority groups must be included in all NIH-supported biomedical and behavioral research projects involving human subjects, unless a clear and compelling rationale and justification establishes that inclusion is inappropriate with respect to the health of the subjects or the purposes of the research.[21]

Research proposals submitted for NIH funding are required to provide detailed information on recruiting and retaining women and minorities, as well as letters of support from community groups with whom the researchers collaborate.

In 2000, the Office of Minority Health (OMH) developed the national standards on the implementation of culturally and linguistically appropriate services (CLAS).[22] CLAS outlines recommendations intended to account for cultural and language preferences in interventions, services, and research. The principal standard is to "provide effective, equitable, understandable, and respectful quality care and services responsive to diverse cultural health beliefs and practices, preferred languages, health literacy, and other communication needs." Other standards are organized into three categories: (a) governance, leadership, and workforce; (b) communication and language assistance; and (c) engagement, continuous improvement, and accountability. The full list of CLAS standards is available on the OMH website (minorityhealth.hhs.gov/omh/browse.aspx?lvl=2&lvlid=53).

Over the past few decades increased attention has been paid to health disparities, but there still remains a need for equitable and culturally competent public health research. Researchers should consider cultural relevance and health equity throughout the research process—from selecting the research topic to disseminating the findings.

Designing a Culturally Competent Public Health Research Study

A culturally competent study begins with identifying key public health research questions with value to the greater society, including minority groups. As discussed in Chapter 2, Literature Search and Research-Question Development, there may be gaps in knowledge and evidence on certain public health research topics because certain populations were excluded in past studies. Equity and contributing to the reduction in health disparities should be key considerations when developing research goals.

Representation of minority populations in public health research is critical to reducing health disparities. However, gaining access to people in these populations and recruiting them for participation in studies can be challenging for several reasons. Unfortunately, past examples of unethical research studies (e.g., Tuskegee syphilis study) created valid and prolonged mistrust in researchers. Historical (and current) biases against groups such as people who identify as transgender create reluctance for research participation. Researchers must acknowledge, understand, and address issues related to reluctance to be involved in studies. Also, the lack of cultural competence in research staff can result in inappropriate and ineffective strategies in communicating with diverse populations. Learning about the people you wish to recruit and retain for your study is paramount. Minority groups can be heterogeneous, and this can impact effective research strategies. Researchers should not assume everyone within a minority group is the same. For example, acculturation can influence differences in racial/ethnic minority groups. A person who is Latinx living in the United States for decades will be different from a person who recently immigrated. Acculturation may also contribute to preferred language, literacy, understanding of customs, and health behaviors—all of which are important research considerations.

Researchers must also think broadly about the social determinants of health, and their impact on minority representation in research. **Social determinants of health** are the conditions in which people live, learn, work, and play that may affect health risks and health outcomes.[23] Lack of transportation, inadequate community resources, unsafe environments, and underperforming schools are all social determinants of health. Researchers need to be aware of these issues and address them throughout the research process. For example, incentives for participation should reflect the needs of the community. Providing childcare at and transportation to intervention sites may bolster participation. Gift cards for internet shopping may be appropriate for the general population, but would not be relevant if participants do not have online access.

Study methodology and analysis are also factors in implementing a culturally competent public health research study. Researchers must ensure data collection tools and strategies are relevant and acceptable to the community. Involving members of the community in development, pilot testing, and implementation can prevent issues related to cultural insensitivity. Data analysis should address the lack of evidence within minority groups. Some research studies may use diverse samples but fail to conduct separate analyses of specific groups. This results in lack of knowledge on specific health risks or intervention effectiveness among minority groups.

The phrase *"nothing about us without us"* exemplifies the ethical importance of community engagement in public health research. A culturally competent study is one in which the community is involved not just as the study population, but is fully integrated into the research process. **Community-based participatory research (CBPR)** is one of the community engagement models commonly used in public health, in which community members and other stakeholders collaborate, share expertise and decision-making throughout all aspects of the research process.[24] CBPR strategies build relationships between researchers and the community in order to create evidence *and* benefit the community.

PRINCIPLES OF COMMUNITY-BASED PARTICIPATORY RESEARCH

- Recognize the community as a unit of identity.
- Identify and build on strengths and resources within a community.
- Facilitate collaborative partnerships in all phases of research.
- Benefit all partners mutually.
- Empower a process to address social inequalities.
- Acknowledge the cyclical and iterative process.
- Address health from an ecological perspective.
- Disseminate findings in relevant ways to all partners.

Source: Isreal BA, Schulz AJ, Parker EA, et.al. Review of community-based research: assessing partnership to improve public health. *Ann Rev Public Health.* 1998;19(1):173–202.[24]

EMERGING ETHICAL ISSUES IN PUBLIC HEALTH RESEARCH

Technological advancements have increased the ways in which researchers can capture, collect, and manage data. Online surveys, Internet interventions, and mobile phone application-based research are common methods used in current public health research. Researchers can even analyze images collected through community cameras streaming content on the Internet.[25] Crowd-sourcing, or having a large number of people provide data, typically over the Internet, is also a novel research method.[25,26] Social media can also be a source of data for public health research.[27] These innovative ways to conduct research require updated guidance for ethical human subjects research. The Collaborative Institutional Training Initiative (CITI), which is the most widely recognized training program for human research protection, includes a module on Internet-based research, but technology advances far quicker than do guidelines or regulations for human subjects research. Privacy and data security are primary ethical concerns with this research. When developing a study, researchers must consider these factors and address them throughout the research process.

PUBLIC HEALTH ETHICS FRAMEWORK AND CODE OF ETHICS

The discipline of public health is deeply embedded in ethical practice and justice. The framework for public health ethics includes three core components, which are all applicable to research.[28] See Box 3.1 for an outline of the framework. This framework outlines considerations for identifying public health issues, evaluating the ethical conflicts, and using this information to choose and justify the best public health option. The Public Health Leadership Society, sponsored by the American Public Health Association, developed the *Principles of the Ethical Practice of Public Health*.[29] These principles comprise the public health code of ethics on which public health is practiced. This code can also be applied to research and is made up of the following components:

- promote health outcomes and preventing disease,
- respect individuals' rights,
- community member input,
- address social determinants of health,
- evidence-based public health,
- community consent,
- timely dissemination of information,
- tailoring for diverse audiences,
- enhance the social and physical environment,
- confidentiality of individual and community information.

BOX 3.1 THE PUBLIC HEALTH ETHICS FRAMEWORK

Analyze the public health issue and context.

> What are the risks and harms of concern?
> What are the public health goals?
> What are the ethical conflicts and competing moral claims of stakeholders?
> Is the source or scope of authority in question?
> Are precedent cases or historical context relevant?
> Do professional codes of ethics provide guidance?

Evaluate and balance the ethical conflicts.

> Balance benefits over harms?
> Are benefits and burdens distributed fairly?
> Can affected groups participate in decisions?
> Are individual choices respected?
> Are professional and civic roles and values respected?

Choose and justify the best public health options.

> What is the effectiveness of the goal? Is the goal likely to be accomplished?
> Are the expected outcomes proportional to the efforts?
> How necessary is the effort?
> Will outcomes by impartial?
> Will intervention have the least infringement?
> Can it be publicly justified?

Source: Data from Public Health Leadership Society, American Public Health Association. *Public Health Leadership Society Principles of the Ethical Practice of Public Health*. 2002. Accessed July 23, 2019. Retrieved from https://www.apha.org/-/media/files/pdf/membergroups/ethics/ethics_brochure.ashx[29]

CHAPTER DISCUSSION QUESTIONS

1. Describe the violations of the principles of the ethical practice of public health in the Tuskegee syphilis study and Havasupai "Diabetes Study." What are ways in which the research could have been conducted to comply with these principles?
2. Identify ways in which you could incorporate principles of CPBR into an intervention study aiming to increase breastfeeding in low-income, African American women.
3. Think about the way in which historical events informed human subjects guidelines and requirements. Since unethical research studies still exist today, how might guidelines and requirements be strengthened?
4. How might an informed-consent document differ in a study on contraception knowledge with adolescents versus adults?
5. How can you improve your knowledge and training in public health research ethics?

RESEARCH PROJECT CHECK-IN

What are the Ethical Considerations for Your Research Project Idea?

Get additional training in research ethics. The CITI training described in this chapter is a useful tool for students and researchers, and is widely accepted as a certification in research ethics. As you progress in the research process, think about the population for your research study idea. Based on the information in this chapter, what are ways to minimize or eliminate any risk to those who participate? Consider the components of informed consent if relevant.

PUBLIC HEALTH RESEARCH METHODS IN REAL LIFE

The Ethics of Community-Based Research

The team was made up of young, motivated researchers who just received funding to assess community residents concerning their perceptions of neighborhood health challenges. They would use the results to implement interventions within the areas identified, which emerged as priorities. Della was excited about this project. She grew up in a similar community and understood the struggles. It was difficult for community members to think about healthy behaviors when many faced unemployment, lack of opportunity, and drug-ridden streets.

The PI of the project was a new professor at the university, and also new to the community, but she was well trained and experienced in community-based research. After meeting with community leaders and holding a forum to explain the project, the team planned to conduct interviews with both formal and informal community leaders. Using the information from these initial interviews, they would then conduct face-to-face surveys at church services and the local library. The PI and all team members were trained and certified to conduct human subjects research as required by their university. The study protocol and data-collection instruments were all approved by the IRB.

Della was an excellent interviewer. The comfort and ease of the participants was apparent as she spoke with them. She connected with the people in the community and was able to obtain thorough and insightful responses to her questions. Based on the interview information, she had significant input in the development of the survey questions. Because of Della and her connection to the community residents, the team exceeded their expected response rate by 10%.

The PI gave Della and the other research assistant the opportunity to conduct the data analysis. They used their biostatistical expertise to run all the significance tests and summarize the results to share with the PI. In the meantime, Della saw a call for abstracts for a local public health conference, for which the theme was challenges to improving social determinants of health. She thought this would be a perfect fit for the results from both the interviews and surveys, but there were only 24 hours left to submit the abstract and her PI was on a transcontinental flight. She made a decision to gather the necessary background information and summarize the findings. Her MPH education made her well versed in abstract writing. She submitted the abstract and met the deadline.

The reviewers of the abstracts for this conference were a mix of public health practitioners and community stakeholders. It just so happened that one of the people interviewed for Della's study, Pastor Stokes, was on the review panel. When he read the abstract, he knew it sounded familiar. When he realized that it was the study in which he participated, he became angry. During the initial community meetings, the residents made it clear that they wanted to hear the results first, before anything was publicized or published. Pastor Stokes felt as if the PI and the research team violated this agreement and disrespected the community residents' wishes.

When the PI of the study found out Della submitted the abstract without her knowledge, she was very disappointed. Not only had the PI just established a relationship with this community, she had hoped for a long-term affiliation as she continued her research at the university. After talking with Pastor Stokes and holding a meeting with community leaders and residents, they agreed that the PI could continue her work there, but insisted on a written agreement of terms. The relationship had been significantly damaged, but not destroyed completely. The PI removed Della from the project, and used the situation as a teachable moment. She required Della attend training on the ethics of community-based research. After Della completed the training and passed the certification test, she was allowed to once again work as a research assistant. Ramifications of the unethical use of community data and further required training prepared Della for future work in communities. She learned undeniably about the sensitivity and ethical considerations of public health research in communities through this experience.

Critical Thinking Questions

1. To what extent do you think Della violated the principles of ethical research? Describe her unethical actions.
2. Did the community have a right to be the first to see the findings? Why was this so important to them?
3. If you were the other research assistant, would you have supported Della's abstract submission? How would you have reacted to her being removed from the project?
4. Do you agree with the way the PI handled Della's actions? Why or why not?
5. How does this type of situation hinder public health research within communities?
6. What are some suggestions for fostering quality community partnerships in research studies?
7. What policies should organizations and universities have in order to ensure ethical research practices in communities?

COUNCIL ON EDUCATION FOR PUBLIC HEALTH ACCREDITATION FOUNDATIONAL KNOWLEDGE AND COMPETENCIES

Foundational Knowledge

Profession and Science of Public Health

- Explain the critical importance of evidence in advancing public health knowledge.

Factors Related to Human Health

- Explain the social, political, and economic determinants of health and how they contribute to population health and health inequities.

Foundational Competencies

Public Health and Healthcare Systems

- Discuss the means by which structural bias, social inequities, and racism undermine health and create challenges to achieving health equity at organizational, community, and societal levels.

Communication

- Describe the importance of cultural competence in communicating public health content.

REFERENCES

1. U.S. Government Printing Office. Electronic code of federal regulations. 2018. Accessed July 19, 2019. https://www.ecfr.gov/cgi-bin/retrieveECFR?gp=&SID=83cd09e1c0f5c6937cd9d7513160fc3f&pitd=20180719&n=pt45.1.46&r=PART&ty=HTML

2. Annas GJ, Grodin MA. Reflections on the 70th anniversary of the Nuremberg doctors' trial. *Am J Public Health*. 2018;108(1):10–12. doi:10.2105/AJPH.2017.304203

3. Centers for Disease Control and Prevention. Tuskegee study. 2017. Accessed July 19, 2019. https://www.cdc.gov/tuskegee/timeline.htm

4. Centers for Disease Control and Prevention. Tuskegee study—presidential apology. 1997. Accessed July 19, 2019. https://www.cdc.gov/tuskegee/clintonp.htm

5. Inter Tribal Council of Arizona. Havasupai tribe: introductory information. 2019. Accessed July 19, 2019. https://itcaonline.com/?page_id=1160

6. Pacheco CM, Daley SM, Brown T, et al. Moving forward: breaking the cycle of mistrust between American Indians and researchers. *Am J Public Health*. 2013;103(12):2152–2159. doi:10.2105/AJPH.2013.301480

7. Drabiak-Syed K. Lessons from Havasupai Tribe v. Arizona State University Board of Regents: recognizing group, cultural, and dignitary harms as legitimate risks warranting integration into research practice. *J Health Biomed Law*. 2010;6(2):175–226.

8. Garrison NA. Genomic justice for Native Americans: impact of the Havasupai Case on genetic research. *Sci Technol Human Values*. 2013;38(2):201–223. doi:10.1177/0162243912470009

9. Arizona Appelate Court. Havasupai tribe of Havasupai reservation v. Arizona Board of Regents. *FindLaw*. 2008. Accessed July 19, 2019. https://caselaw.findlaw.com/az-court-of-appeals/1425062.html

10. United States Library of Congress. *Trials of War Criminals before the Nuremberg Military Tribunals under Control Council Law No. 10*. Vol. 2. Washington, DC: U.S. Government Printing Office; 1949:181–182.

11. World Medical Association. Declaration of Helsinki–ethical principles for medical research involving human subjects. 2013. Accessed July 19, 2019. https://www.wma.net/policies-post/wma-declaration-of-helsinki-ethical-principles-for-medical-research-involving-human-subjects

12. U.S. Department of Health and Human Services. Read the Belmont report. 1979. Accessed July 19, 2019. https://www.hhs.gov/ohrp/regulations-and-policy/belmont-report/read-the-belmont-report/index.html

13. Lawson G, Schapiro R. Amendment X—the United States constitution. Amendment X: common interpretation. 2018. Accessed July 22, 2019. https://constitutioncenter.org/interactive-constitution/amendments/amendment-x

14. Research Office of Oregon State University. Cannabis research. 2019. Accessed July 22, 2019. https://research.oregonstate.edu/cannabis-research

15. U.S. Department of Health and Human Services. Informed consent FAQs. 2019. Accessed July 22, 2019. https://www.hhs.gov/ohrp/regulations-and-policy/guidance/faq/informed-consent/index.html

16. U.S. Department of Health and Human Services. Health information privacy: research. 2018. Accessed July 22, 2019. https://www.hhs.gov/hipaa/for-professionals/special-topics/research/index.html

17. McCambridge J, Kypri K, Bendtsen P, et al. The use of deception in public health behavioral intervention trials: a case study of three online alcohol trials. *Am J Bioeth*. 2013;13(11):39. doi:10.1080/15265161.2013.839751

18. Zutlevics T. Could providing financial incentives to research participants be ultimately self-defeating? *Res Ethics*. 2016;12(3):137–148. doi:10.1177/1747016115626756

19. Office of Minority Health. National CLAS standards. Cultural competency. 2000. Accessed July 23, 2019. https://minorityhealth.hhs.gov/omh/browse.aspx?lvl=2&lvlid=53

20. Pinn VW. Achieving diversity and its benefits in clinical research. *AMA J Ethics*. 2004;6(12):561–565. doi:10.1001/virtualmentor.2004.6.12.pfor2-0412

21. National Institutes of Health. NIH guide: NIH guidelines on the inclusion of women and minorities as subjects in clinical research. 1994. Accessed July 23, 2019. https://grants.nih.gov/grants/guide/notice-files/not94-100.html

22. Samuel-Hodge CD, Johnson CM, Braxton DF, et al. Effectiveness of diabetes prevention program translations among African Americans. *Obes Rev*. 2014;15(suppl 4):107–124. doi:10.1111/obr.12211

23. Centers for Disease Control and Prevention. Social determinants of health: know what affects health. 2018. Accessed July 24, 2019. https://www.cdc.gov/socialdeterminants/index.htm.

24. Israel BA, Schulz AJ, Parker EA, et al. Review of community-based research: assessing partnership approaches to improve public health. *Annu Rev Public Health*. 1998;19(1):173–202. doi:10.1146/annurev.publhealth.19.1.173

25. Hipp JA, Adlakha D, Eyler AA, et al. Emerging technologies: webcams and crowd-sourcing to identify active transportation. *Am J Prev Med*. 2013;44(1):96–97. doi:10.1016/j.amepre.2012.09.051

26. World Health Organization. Crowdsourcing in health and health research: a practical guide. 2018. Accessed July 23, 2019. https://apps.who.int/iris/bitstream/handle/10665/273039/TDR-STRA-18.4-eng.pdf?ua=1

27. Pagoto S, Nebeker C. How scientists can take the lead in establishing ethical practices for social media research. *J Am Med Inform Assoc*. 2019;26(4):311–313. doi:10.1093/jamia/ocy174

28. Kass NE. An ethics framework for public health. *Am J Public Health*. 2001;91(11):1776–1782. doi:10.2105/AJPH.91.11.1776

29. Public Health Leadership Society, American Public Health Association. Public health leadership society principles of the ethical practice of public health. 2002. Accessed July 23, 2019. https://www.apha.org/-/media/files/pdf/membergroups/ethics/ethics_brochure.ashx

30. Milgram S. *Obedience to Authority: An Experimental View*. New York, NY: Harper & Row Publishers; 1974.

ADDITIONAL READINGS AND RESOURCES

MacQueen KM, Buehler JW. Ethics, practice and research in public health. *Am J Public Health*. 2004;94(6):928–931. doi:10.2105/AJPH.94.6.928

Public Health Leadership Society, American Public Health Association. Principles of the ethical practice of public health. 2002. Accessed July 19, 2019. https://www.apha.org/-/media/files/pdf/membergroups/ethics/ethics_brochure.ashx

Sanders Thompson V, Hood S. Community based participatory research. In: Goodman MS, Sanders Thompson V, eds. *Public Health Research Methods for Partnerships and Practice*. New York , NY: CRC Press; 2018:2–22.

Special Anniversary Issue: Focus on History. *Am J Public Health*. 1997;87(11).

U.S. Department of Health and Human Services. Office for Human Research Protections. 2019. Accessed July 19, 2019. https://www.hhs.gov/ohrp/about-ohrp/index.html

II

RESEARCH DETAILS AND DESIGN

This section gets deeper into the specifics of planning public health research. Once you identify your research topic and question, you will need to create definitions of relevant concepts and figure out the best ways to measure them. Chapter 4 outlines the importance of operationalization and measurement, and how this step in the research process impacts the rest of the research project. Chapter 5 describes the significance of sampling in research, and provides examples of strategies commonly used in public health research. Chapters 6 and 7 explain causality in research and the impact of study designs on this concept. Many different study designs, along with the advantages and disadvantages of each of them are described. Chapter 8 is all about budgeting for research. It outlines some of the main funders of public health research, and provides information on how to develop and justify a research budget for a project proposal.

Operationalization and Measurement

What gets measured gets improved.
　　—Peter Drucker, business management consultant

LEARNING OBJECTIVES

After reading this chapter, the reader will be able to

- Understand the importance of operationalization in research.
- Develop quality hypotheses.
- Define different types of research variables and the ways in which they interact.
- Explain the concepts of internal validity and reliability.
- Develop a conceptual model.

INTRODUCTION

Good science is based on measurement. Think back to your elementary school science experiments. Planting seeds and varying their exposure to factors, such as light or water, is a common assignment. The young scientist measures the growth and takes notes on other aspects of the plant, while also keeping track of hours of daylight. When the experiment is complete, the data (height of plant, hours exposed) informs the conclusion. This elementary lesson is good example of how research relies on data, and data has to be measured.

Many public health issues are complex, and measuring or quantifying them can be challenging. For example, how might you measure "good" health? What does "good" health look like? There are many definitions of "health," but what is considered "good" needs a more explicit definition in order to be measured. Maybe good health can be defined as no missed work or school days or normal biomarkers in age-appropriate preventive screening. How you choose to define good health should be rooted in past literature, relevant to your study population, and consistent with your research goals. Some public health topics are more tangible to measure, but still broad in scope. Suppose you are interested in studying the topic of smoking. How will you define smoking behavior? Whether a person currently smokes? Has ever smoked? Smokes only a certain amount per day? Uses electronic cigarettes? Defining your topic is an important step in the research process.

The literature search and development of the research question clarify the concept you wish to study. Conceptualization leads to the next step, operationalization. **Operationalization** is the development of specific definitions for all relevant factors related to the topic of interest. Operationalization turns vague or ambiguous concepts into detailed descriptions, which can be measured. In order to operationalize, a researcher needs to identify indicators logically related to the concept of interest. These indicators inform the development of study variables (Table 4.1). Operationalization means different things in quantitative versus qualitative research. Although it is still important to define concepts in qualitative studies, the quantitative measures require more precision and objective operationalization. Chapter 11, Qualitative Study Designs, further explores qualitative operationalization.

VARIABLES IN RESEARCH

Operational definitions lead to the development of variables. In research, **variables** are defined as anything that can "vary" or has different values. Variables should be well defined

TABLE 4.1 EXAMPLES OF OPERATIONALIZING CONCEPTS INTO VARIABLES

Concept ⟶	Operationalization ⟶	Variables
Walking	Walking for activity Walking for transportation	Steps per day Location of walking
Social media	Computer or mobile use of social media platforms	Time per day Sites used
High BP management	Participation in an evidence-based program BP in health range	Number of classes attended BP measurements
Effectiveness of worksite wellness program	Absenteeism Reduced healthcare costs	Number of days missed Healthcare claims totals

BP, blood pressure.

and feasible to observe or measure. They can be persons, things, behaviors, or situations having different qualities or quantities. These differences are called **attributes** (Figure 4.1). Think about education as an example. You can divide this variable into two attributes (e.g., high school graduate, not a high school graduate) or you could choose to use more specific attributes (e.g., some high school, high school graduate, some college, college graduate). The way in which you categorize variable attributes should be consistent with theoretical or logical groups relating to your research question. Keep in mind that the lowest number of attributes a variable can have and still be "variable" is two.

Quantitative research studies aim to identify the influence of one variable on the next. Researchers capture the direction of the influence by designating independent and dependent variables. In general terms, the **independent variable** (IV) is the one presumed to influence or cause the **dependent variable** (DV). In a study of sociodemographics and intent to breastfeed in pregnant women, intent to breastfeed would be the DV, whereas factors, such as age, race/ethnicity, and education, would be the IVs. If assessing the effectiveness of a weight-loss intervention, weight loss would be the DV and program factors, such as attendance and engagement, would be IVs. Identifying IV and DV is essential to developing research hypotheses for quantitative studies.

Sometimes research is not just a neat and tidy depiction of IV influence on the DV. Additional variables may affect the IV–DV relationship through mediation or moderation (Figure 4.2). A **mediating variable** (sometimes called intervening variable) is something that influences the mechanism by which the IV affects a DV. A mediating variable may be a factor in *why* the IV–DV relationship exists in the first place. If we think our intervention increases fruit and vegetable consumption by first increasing awareness of places to

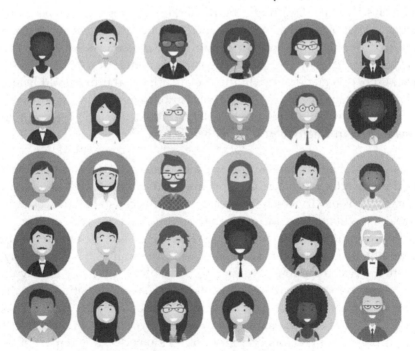

FIGURE 4.1 **What are examples of variables and attributes you see in this figure?**

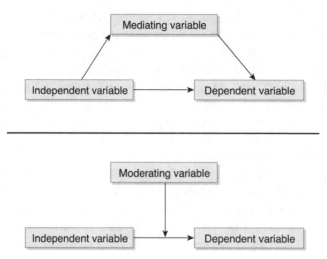

FIGURE 4.2 **Diagram illustrating mediating and moderating variables.**

purchase food, this awareness would be considered a mediating variable. When you fully account for the effect of the mediating variable, the relationship between the IV and DV might not exist. **Moderating variables** influence the strength or direction of the IV–DV relationship, and contextualize the effect between the IV and DV. Including moderating variables in your study may help answer the questions: Whom does it work for? Under what conditions? At what times? For example, the relationship between social support (IV) and perceived health (DV) might be moderated by gender. Maybe there will be a lower or higher effect of social support on perceived health in men compared to women. A good way to differentiate between mediating and moderating variables is to identify whether the independent variable causes the variable in question. If yes, then the variable is mediating; if no, it is moderating. In the social support and perceived health example, does social support cause gender? The answer is no, so gender is a moderating variable. In the example of increasing fruit and vegetable intake, does the intervention cause an increased awareness in where to purchase healthy food? Yes, so awareness is a mediating variable.

There are additional variables in research that are accounted for in different ways. Controlling for the effects of variables is common in public health research studies. A **controlled variable** is one in which the researcher holds constant balances across groups, or neutralizes so it will not have an effect on the study. Suppose you conduct two sessions of the same 4-week immunization intervention to increase vaccine uptake; the first session in January, and the second in February. The session chosen by participants may confound the relationship between the intervention (IV) and uptake (DV) so you may use "session attended" as a control variable. A **constant variable** has no variation. It is the same for all cases in a study, and helps control the effects of that variable. If you choose to only include people living in one zip code as your sample, you rule out any effect that might occur due to differences in factors present in other zip codes. It is important to note that defining controlled or constant variables should be theory or logic based, and relevant to the research question. What may be controlled for or held constant in one study could potentially be an IV in another study.

RELATIONSHIP AMONG VARIABLES

A correlation is a relationship between variables, but does not imply one variable caused the other. Correlations can be positive, negative, or curvilinear (Figure 4.3). In a **positive correlation**, the value of the DV increases or decreases in the same direction as the IV. In other words, they both go up or they both go down. For example, as number of years of smoking cigarettes

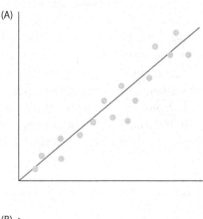

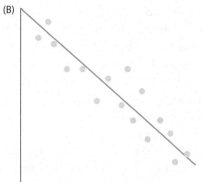

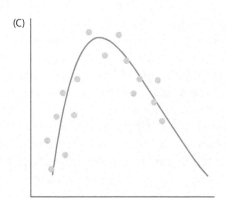

FIGURE 4.3 **Depictions of relationships between variables. (A) Positive correlation: Both variables either go up or down. (B) Negative correlation: One variable goes up and the other goes down. (C) Curvilinear relationship: Both variables go up or down together, then at some point they diverge into opposite directions.**

increases, the risk of lung cancer increases. In this case, both variables rise. If stress levels are reduced, participants miss fewer days of work. Both stress level and days missed decrease. These are two examples of positive correlations. A **negative correlation** is one in which the variables change in opposite directions. One of the variables increases as the other decreases. If an older adult increases muscle strength, the chance for injuries from falling decreases. Another example of a negative correlation: When engagement in evidence-based diabetes prevention programs increases, the prevalence of diabetes onset decreases. Relationships between variables can also be more complex than a straight increase or decrease. **Curvilinear correlations** occur when the relationship between the variables transforms at certain variable levels. For example, in an 8-week tobacco-cessation intervention delivered via text message, you notice engagement decreases in the first 4 weeks, then increases over the remaining 4 weeks. This represents a curvilinear relationship between the intervention (IV) and the engagement (DV), and data would plot in a U-shape. The relationship would also be curvilinear if engagement increased in the first 4 weeks, and then decreased over the course of the remaining intervention, resulting in the data fitting an upside down U-shape.

CONCEPTUAL FRAMEWORK AND HYPOTHESIS DEVELOPMENT

A **conceptual framework** outlines the theoretical or logical relationships among variables, and the progression from the IV to the DV. In a conceptual framework, the concepts and associated variables are organized and linked sequentially. These frameworks are typically based on theory, evidence, or specific knowledge. Developing a conceptual framework is useful for considering proposed causal linkages between the variables in the study and other key factors potentially influencing the outcome (e.g., moderating variables). They are also a good way to summarize and integrate salient factors from relevant theories and literature on the topic.

When developing a conceptual framework, start with the end point and work backwards to identify the potential relationships among the variables. If the outcome you wish to measure in your study is the teen pregnancy rate, then this would be the end point, which is placed to the far right of your model (if horizontal) and at the bottom (if vertical). See Figure 4.4 for an example of a conceptual framework on factors affecting walking behavior in a rural community. In this example, the program goals or outcomes are improvements in physical activity, walking, and body mass.

The next step in developing a conceptual framework is to identify potential correlates of the outcome of interest based on theory or other studies. Think specifically about how the concepts will be operationalized and measured. Use arrows to identify causal relationships and directionality between concepts. The proposed relationships between the concepts in the framework inform the development of the research hypothesis. The process of developing a conceptual framework is as valuable as the completed product. It helps the researcher think broadly about the proposed study, and formulate a detailed model to inform the next steps in the research process.

Hypotheses are statements that predict the nature and extent of relationships between variables based on your research question or research goals in quantitative studies. The proposed relationships in hypotheses can be based on theory, limited evidence, or innovative ideas about the way in which variables may interact. Crafting well-thought-out hypotheses is key to quality research. Good hypotheses are specific, measurable, and stated in a such a way that they can be accepted or rejected. Many studies include more than one hypothesis, as there

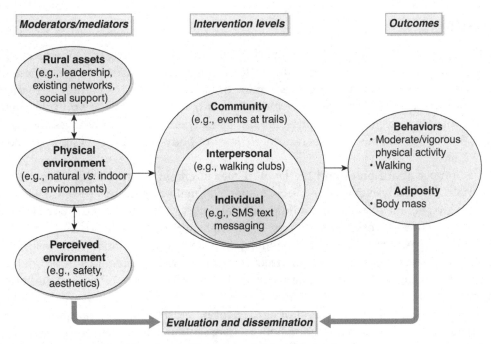

FIGURE 4.4 **Example of a conceptual framework.**
Source: Beck, A.M., Eyler, A.A., Hipp, A., et al. A multilevel approach for promoting physical activity in rural communities: a cluster randomized controlled trial. *BMC Public Health.* 2019;19:126.[3]

are several different types. The **null hypothesis** states that there no differences in attributes, effect, or relation between variables. "There is no difference in weight lost between women who complete Intervention A versus Intervention B" is an example of a null hypothesis. An **alternative hypothesis** affirms the existence of differences in attributes, effect, or relationship between variables. An alternative hypothesis to the previous example could be stated, "Women completing Intervention A will lose more weight than women who complete Intervention B." Hypotheses can be directional or nondirectional (i.e., will increase or decrease), causal (i.e., will have greater or less), or associative (there is a positive relationship between). Prior research studies may inform the best ways to present the alternative hypothesis.

The results from hypothesis testing are important beyond an individual study. Other researchers can test the same hypotheses to build evidence for public health programs, policies, and interventions. Even when the study results do not support the hypothesis, the information is valuable to the field. This creates an opportunity to suggest ways the concept or topic can be explored in future studies.

A good hypothesis...
- is based on your research question,
- predicts the outcome of your research,
- is directly related to the variables of interest,
- is clear and concise, and
- is testable.

MEASUREMENT

Variable types can differ by the number and characteristics of attributes, and the way in which you operationalize them plays an important role in quantitative measurement. Variables with only two attributes (e.g., completing intervention or not completing intervention) are **dichotomous, or binary**. When variables have more than two attributes, they are **polychotomous**. The attributes in polychotomous variables can be categorical (e.g., body mass index: <25, 25–29.9, 30+) or continuous (e.g., each numeric level of body mass index is an attribute: 25, 25.1, 25.2, etc.).

The number of attributes and the **level of measurement** are fundamental to selecting appropriate data-analysis methods. (See Chapter 11, Qualitative Study Designs.) There are four basic levels of measurement: nominal, ordinal, interval, and ratio. In the **nominal** level, attributes are "named" or categorized by some characteristic. Characterizing type of diet into omnivore, pescatarian, vegetarian, and vegan is an example of nominal measurement. In the **ordinal** level, categories are "ordered" in some way. The categories in ordinal measurement are arranged in order of magnitude of the characteristic, but the intervals between the numbers are not equal. We may know whether one is less or more, but we do not know by how much. Scales indicating level of agreement or satisfaction are examples of ordinal measurement. For example, satisfaction with an intervention could be measured using "very satisfied, satisfied, unsatisfied, and very unsatisfied." With this scale, the exact value of the increments between each choice is unknown. **Interval** level of measurement includes both an order and equal intervals between scale values. However, interval scales do not have a true zero. An example of an interval scale is temperature measured in Fahrenheit or Celsius. In both of these scales, zero is arbitrary; 0 °F and 0 °C do not indicate an absence of temperature. **Ratio** measurements have order, equal intervals, and a true zero. The difference between the intervals is always measured from a zero point. Variables measured on a ratio scale can be used for mathematical equations. An example of a ratio variable is income. A person who earns $60,000 per year makes two times as much as someone earning $30,000 per year, and six times as much as someone earning $10,000 per year. See Table 4.2 for more examples of levels of measurement.

The goal of measurement is to accurately represent the concept you are trying to measure. However, the measurement process is vulnerable and measurement errors may occur. Measurement errors are inaccuracies stemming from either systematic or random sources. **Systematic error** reflects an imprecise measure due to the way data were collected or factors related to those who provided the data. Biases in data collection can cause systematic error. A **bias** is a misrepresentation in measurement due to personal views or beliefs, and it affects the way people answer questions thereby distorting true responses. A common reason for systematic error due to bias is **social desirability**: people tend to answer questions in a way they think is socially acceptable. The risk for social desirability in responses increases with the sensitivity of topics being researched. A high school student may underreport alcohol consumption because they are not of legal drinking age. A person may also overreport behaviors that are more socially desirable, such as healthy eating or physical activity. Sometimes the process of data collection impacts social desirability. If a person knows their responses will be connected to their identity, their answers may be biased by social desirability more so than if the data were collected anonymously. Social desirability can also result in **acquiescent response set bias,** or agreeing or disagreeing with all statements in order to provide what one thinks to be favorable responses. Acquiescent response set bias is a source of systematic error.

TABLE 4.2 LEVELS OF MEASUREMENT

Type	Definition	Example
Nominal	Categories with no numerical value	What type of healthcare provider do you see on a regular basis? **1.** Physician **2.** Physician's assistant **3.** Nurse practitioner **4.** Nurse **5.** Other
Ordinal	Scale in which each value is rank ordered in a way that is higher or lower than the previous value, but intervals are unknown or not equal	How satisfied are you with the diabetes-prevention program? **1.** Very satisfied **2.** Somewhat satisfied **3.** Neutral **4.** Somewhat unsatisfied **5.** Unsatisfied
Interval	Scale in which values have order and equal intervals, without a true zero point	What was your ACT score? _____
Ratio	Scale in which values have order and equal intervals, with a true zero point	What was the change (in inches) of your hamstring flexibility? **1.** 0 inches **2.** 1 inch **3.** 2 inches **4.** 3 inches **5.** 4 inches

ACT, American College Testing

Responses may overestimate or underestimate true values in unpredictable ways, resulting in random error. **Random errors** are due to chance and have no consistent pattern. Sometimes factors such as mood or circumstance influence responses. Imagine filling out a survey on level of anxiety after being involved in a minor car crash the day of data collection. Your responses might be different than if you were more calm and relaxed. Random error may also be due to other conditions. Factors such as noise, lighting, and temperature may cause distorted responses.

Two criteria for evaluating the quality of measurement procedures are reliability and validity. **Reliability** means the degree of consistency something has. The more reliable a measure is, the less likely it is to be impacted by random error. If you were measuring a phenomenon that is not changing, you would expect that repeating a measure would yield the same results. A reliable scale would report the same weight if the same person steps on it once, steps off, then steps on it again. However, consistency of measurement does not guarantee accuracy. Although the scale records the same weight upon repeated measures, it is not an indication the scale provides an accurate weight.

There are several different types of reliability. **Test–retest reliability** is a measure of stability over time. Administering an instrument to collect data from a sample of people, then having those same people complete the same measure again is a way to assess test–retest reliability. Comparing the scores from one time to the next will provide an indication of the measure's stability. Seven to 14 days between tests is a time frame commonly used in public health, but best practices for the amount of time between the first data collection and the second varies by construct. Look to past methods in the literature on the topic of the research for recommendations.

Another type of reliability is **internal consistency reliability**. The items throughout a measure should be consistent, whereby answers to questions relating to similar concepts should be highly associated with one another. For example, if respondents expressed agreement with the statements "I like to ride bicycles" and "I've enjoyed riding bicycles in the past," and disagreement with the statement "I hate riding bicycles," this would be indicative of good internal consistency. An example of a statistic commonly used to measure internal consistency reliability is Cronbach's alpha coefficient. This score is a calculation of all possible ways to divide a scale in half to figure the correlation of the test within itself. Statistical software can quickly compute this score, and acceptable values of alpha range from 0.70 to 0.95.[1]

The degree of agreement or consistency among multiple observers is called **inter-rater reliability**. If your research team is tasked with assessing physical activity in children on an elementary-school playground, each observation needs to accurately reflect the actual activity. Quantitative counts or qualitative observations of the same time and place should result in the same data. When comparing observations from two researchers, the data should be mostly consistent. Acceptable levels of agreement among observations can range from 70% to 90%.[2] Explicitly operationalizing constructs and providing observer training are two ways to enhance inter-rater reliability.

A consistent and reliable assessment tool is only half of the quality-measurement equation. A measure must also be valid. **Validity** refers to the extent to which a measure is a true reflection or real meaning of the concept it is intended to measure. Types of validity range from general to more specific. In a general sense, **face validity** is a subjective judgment of whether a measure is a reasonable way to measure some concept or if a logical relationship between the variable and the proposed measure exists. For example, it makes sense to assess mathematical ability by using a set of math problems. Content validity goes a bit more indepth than face validity. **Content validity** is the degree to which a measure covers an entire concept. Simple addition problems do not cover the range of mathematical ability, so an assessment solely including addition problems would not have high content validity for measuring mathematical ability. This is particularly important for complex public health issues. For example, an assessment of tobacco-control efforts would need to encompass a broad range of factors such as tobacco taxes, clean indoor air policies, sales restrictions, and so on. A measure with high content validity includes an adequate sample of all the elements of the concept being measured.

Criterion validity means scores on one measure are similar to scores on another measure of the same condition or criterion. There are two types of criterion validity. **Predictive validity** occurs when scores on one measure can *predict* the scores on a similar measure.

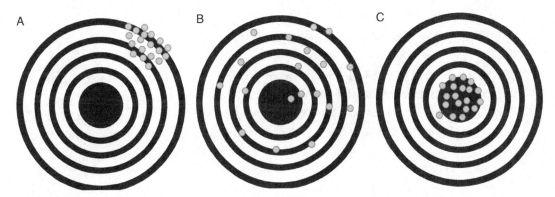

FIGURE 4.5 Visual depictions of validity and reliability. (A) Reliable, but not valid; the repeated measures result in consistency, but the data is not in the target of the concept being studied. (B) Neither reliable (measures not consistent), nor valid (misses the mark most times). (C) Both reliable (consistent time after time) and valid (accurately depicts target concept).

A high score on an aerobic fitness assessment would likely predict a high-score frequency and intensity of exercise. **Concurrent validity** is a type of criterion validity that exists when scores on one measure are closely related to scores on another measure. For example, outcomes of assessments on stress and coping skills would likely be concurrent, or concomitant. Past literature on the research topic of interest can reveal options for comparative measures.

The best quantitative measures are reliable and valid. Although reliability is a precursor to validity, reliability does not ensure validity. You could have a measure that is consistent from one time to the next, but be highly inaccurate in measuring the intended concept. A common depiction of the relationship between reliability and validity is the bull's eye. As shown in Figure 4.5, each dot represents a score from the same measure in a research study. The middle of the bull's eye represents the precise concept. The first of the three bull's eyes shows results closely clustered, but off the mark. The responses fall into a consistent pattern and are reliable, but if the center is the accurate measure of the concept, the measure is not valid. The second figure shows the results dotted all over the bull's eye in an unreliable and inconsistent pattern, and outside of the center circle. This measure is neither valid nor reliable. The third figure depicts the ideal validity and reliability. The results are clustered and located in the center. A valid and reliable measure will increase the likelihood for quality results and reduce the measurement error.

Well-operationalized concepts along with valid and reliable ways to measure them can be achieved with careful preparation. Consider the following in this phase of the research process:

- Look to past studies for ideas on operationalizing variables and conceptual models.
- Include members of the population of interest to provide feedback on appropriateness of definitions and conceptual model.
- Refer to best practices for reducing measurement error.
- Use existing valid and reliable measures if possible.
- Keep track of the process of operationalization. Notes will be helpful when writing a research report.

CHAPTER DISCUSSION QUESTIONS

1. Why is it important to clearly define the variables you aim to use in your research study?
2. Why is developing a conceptual model an important step in research-study planning?
3. What factors would you consider in developing hypotheses for your study on racial/ethnic differences in vaping? Create at least three different hypotheses for this hypothetical study.
4. Discuss ways to ensure internal validity for a measure of work stress among nurses.

RESEARCH PROJECT CHECK-IN

How Will You Define and Assess?

Public health topics are complex, and there are many different ways to describe and define related factors. Make a list of concepts associated to your research question or study aim. Take the time to develop a conceptual framework. The process of developing this framework will help you make connections among different components of your study. Include specific definitions of variables, and begin to plan for ways to address reliability and validity. Check back with the literature to get a sense of how other researchers might have framed similar topics of study.

PUBLIC HEALTH RESEARCH METHODS IN REAL LIFE

Define and Conquer

Regina was a program evaluator who was recently hired to develop an evaluation plan for a public health intervention. The intervention aimed to test strategies to increase the awareness of the importance of the flu vaccine and uptake of a free flu vaccine at a clinic situated between two large worksites (Worksite A and Worksite B). The target population of the intervention was employees who worked in the building adjacent to the clinic. The researchers planned to compare the effectiveness of emails from the human resource department in Worksite A with emails plus flyers in bathrooms in Worksite B. The hypothesis was that the combination of methods would be more effective at increasing awareness and vaccine rates than emails alone.

The main outcome would be easy to define for the evaluation. Did the number of vaccines given to employees increase? Were the numbers of those vaccinated different by worksite? But Regina wondered how to measure the other factors. How would they define "increased awareness"? Did it mean learning the flu was a significant health risk? Did it mean seeing (and reading) the emails and bathroom flyers? The people they assess should be aware of the importance of getting the vaccine, too. How would this be defined?

There were so many components to think about. It was beneficial that the intervention team had already developed a conceptual model. The model described theoretical and conceptual factors that might influence the outcome. Regina decided to start with the model to help operationalize the components important to the evaluation plan. First step: Define the variables and make sure they are measurable. She decided to look at effectiveness in two different ways. First, assess the prevalence of flu vaccine uptake for employees of both worksites and compare these to last year's vaccine rates. Second, compare the rates at posttest between the two worksites.

Awareness was the more difficult concept to operationalize. She decided to define awareness at three levels. The lowest level of awareness would be defined as having seen the flyers or emails about the free flu vaccines at the clinic. The next level of awareness was defined as having seen the flyers and/or emails and remembering at least one fact about the flu vaccine that was presented as content in the emails and/or flyers. The third level of awareness was having seen the emails and/or flyers, remembering one fact about the flu vaccine, and getting the vaccine at the clinic. These three levels would be assessed and compared for each worksite.

Regina looked to the literature for valid and reliable surveys to use, and she found one appropriate for the characteristics of the population and the study setting. She made a plan to identify vaccine rates of employees at the worksites through their worksite wellness survey data. Although not every employee filled out the survey, it had a response rate of 68% at Worksite A and 72% at Worksite B. She made a note that this was self-reported, and might reflect a bias when compared to actual number of vaccines given. Regina also was aware of the timing of the intervention. She wanted to make sure to collect baseline information on flu awareness at least 3 weeks before the clinic started to give the vaccines. Postintervention data would be collected 16 weeks after the baseline data collection.

Her hard work in operationalizing the variables paid off. The detailed evaluation plan was well received by the research team, and Regina looked forward to conquering the evaluation.

Critical Thinking Questions

1. Why is it often difficult to define *awareness*? How would you define *awareness* in this scenario?
2. *Operationalization* means the variables need to be measurable. How else might effectiveness of this intervention be measured?
3. What factors need to be considered when comparing the two worksite populations?
4. What if, during the intervention, several people in Worksite A were hospitalized with the flu?
5. How would Regina make sure the assessments were culturally appropriate for the employee groups?
6. How would you identify mediating and moderating factors of vaccine uptake for this group? How might this impact the measure of outcome effectiveness?

COUNCIL ON EDUCATION FOR PUBLIC HEALTH FOUNDATIONAL KNOWLEDGE AND COMPETENCIES

Foundational Knowledge

Profession and Science of Public Health

- Explain the critical importance of evidence in advancing public health knowledge.

Foundational Competencies

Evidence-Based Approaches to Public Health

- Select quantitative and qualitative data-collection methods appropriate for a given public health context.

Planning and Management to Promote Health

- Assess population needs, assets, and capabilities that affect communities' health.
- Select methods to evaluate public health programs

REFERENCES

1. Tavakol M, Dennick R. Making sense of Cronbach's alpha. *Int J Med Educ.* 2011;2:53–55. doi:10.5116/ijme.4dfb.8dfd

2. Cohen JA. A coefficient of agreement for nominal scales. *Educ Psychol Meas.* 1960;20:37–46.

3. Beck, A.M., Eyler, A.A., Hipp, A., et al. A multilevel approach for promoting physical activity in rural communities: a cluster randomized controlled trial. *BMC Public Health.* 2019;19:126.

ADDITIONAL READINGS AND RESOURCES

Association of State and Territorial Health Officials. Operationalizing tobacco cessation policy efforts. 2019. Accessed July 15, 2019. Audio podcast available at https://www.astho.org/generickey/GenericKeyDetails.aspx?contentid=21587&folderid=5158&catid=7237

Centers for Disease Control and Prevention. Health-related quality of life (HRQOL): Measurement properties, validity, reliability, and responsiveness. n.d. Updated October 31, 2018. Accessed July 15, 2019. https://www.cdc.gov/hrqol/measurement.htm

Paradies Y, Stevens M. Conceptual diagrams in public health research. *J Epidemiol Community Health.* 2005;59(12):1012–1013. doi:10.1136/jech.2005.036913

Pedersen SJ, Kitic CM, Bird ML, et al. Is self-reporting workplace activity worthwhile? Validity and reliability of occupational sitting and physical activity questionnaire in desk-based workers. *BMC Public Health.* 2016;16:836. https://bmcpublichealth.biomedcentral.com/articles/10.1186/s12889-016-3537-4

Voetsch K, Sequeria S, Holmes Chavez A. A customizable model for chronic disease coordination: Lessons learned from the coordinated chronic disease program. *Prev Chronic Dis.* 2016;13:150509. doi:10.5888/pcd13.150509

Sampling

Sampling should be designed to guard against unplanned selectiveness.
　　—American Association of Public Opinion Research,
　　　　　　　Best Practices for Survey Research

LEARNING OBJECTIVES

After reading this chapter, the reader will be able to

- Define sampling.
- Differentiate between probability and nonprobability sampling methods.
- Identify the advantages and disadvantages of sampling methods.
- Understand sampling error.
- Identify considerations for selecting sampling methods.

INTRODUCTION

Sampling food in a grocery store or ordering a sampler platter in a restaurant is quite different than sampling in research. **Sampling** is an examination of a portion of a larger group of people, places, or things in a research study, then applying the results to the larger population. Simply put, a part of the population is studied to gain information on the whole population. In many instances, it would not be feasible to gather data from every single person or factor of interest. Imagine the time and resources needed to gather data from every parent in the United States who chose to immunize their child with the human papillomavirus (HPV) vaccine in 2018. Getting data from a sample of parents is more feasible. If done correctly, the results from the sample would reflect the whole population of parents. We often think of "people" as the population, but sampling can apply to places such as schools, clinics, or cities. If you want to study fresh food availability in urban areas, you could choose a sample of cities to study rather than collecting data on every store in every city or metropolitan area. Samples in public health research can also be "things." You could sample policies, documents, or media articles. If you want to measure the extent to which news stories on the opioid crisis mention mental health services, you do not have to search for and analyze every single article. Your time and effort would be better spent finding and analyzing a representative sample of articles. Whatever your study targets are, a quality sample adds rigor and generalizability to your study.

Sampling in public health research is not a new concept. In 1954, Woolsey et al. published a paper in the *American Journal of Public Health* on the broad applications of sampling in the field of public health.[1] Sampling can be used for:

- information such as demographics or health characteristics for program planning
- pilot testing interventions or programs
- evaluation of interventions or programs
- environmental health surveys
- measurement of healthcare access
- summaries of health issues
- communication of vital statistics
- system evaluation, such as those used in recording birth and death records

Generalizability of research findings helps build evidence for effective public health practice. Results from a study conducted with an appropriate sample increase the likelihood that the findings apply to the larger population accurately. Sampling may also influence the extent to which results can be generalized to other, different populations. This broad generalization of results beyond the context of the study is called **external validity**. As stated in Chapter 1, The Importance of Research in Public Health, research builds evidence, and the better we can apply findings within and across study populations, the more effective our public health efforts will be.

Sampling discussed in this chapter applies to quantitative studies. The sampling methods for qualitative studies differ, and are discussed in detail in Chapter 11, Qualitative Study Designs. However, whether you are doing a quantitative study or a qualitative study, your choice in sampling method should relate to your research questions and study objectives. Theories guiding your research topic can also influence sampling strategies. Practicality is another factor to consider when deciding about sample selection. The time frame available for the study and the cost of collecting data may limit sampling options. Researchers should also consider their ability to access their population of interest. Some researchers use previously created lists to frame their sample. For example, the U.S. Census provides many types of lists useful in sampling. The National Center for Education Statistics (NCES) collects data on all school districts in the United States. Information included in the publicly available NCES list includes district office addresses and demographic characteristics. Researchers interested in U.S. schools might opt to use this list to develop their sample. Regulatory organizations may also have list information from entities required to be licensed or registered. These may be available to the public or available by request. For example, the Colorado Department of Human Services, Division of Children and Families maintains a database of licensed child-care centers within the state. If you are interested in assessing policies or practices in child-care within Colorado, this list might be helpful in identifying your sample. The availability of preexisting lists enhances the accessibility to sample populations. When contemplating using lists for sampling, researchers should always investigate the parameters of the lists and how they are maintained or updated. Even the most current lists can include duplicates, invalid cases, or inaccurate contacts. They all need to be factored into the sampling plan.

There are ethical considerations to sampling for public health research. Sometimes hard-to-reach people are omitted from the sample. If full representation is needed to answer your research question, all populations need to be included. There are disparities in cell phone, smartphone, and computer ownership in the United States. If email addresses or cell phone numbers are used to determine your sample, not every person has an equal chance of being selected. Just as in operationalization and measurement, involving members of the community you wish to study in the planning phases can inform the most ethical and relevant sample strategy.

THE SAMPLING PROCESS

The first step in the sampling process is to revisit the purpose of your research. What type of sample do you need to be successful in answering your research questions or achieving your research objectives? Determining this helps you outline your population. Think about the sampling process as going from large to small. The **population** (sometimes called *theoretical population*) is the entire set of people, places, or things to which you will generalize results. The population is made up of **elements** (individual units). In some studies, the whole population is used as the sample. This is only feasible if the whole population is small (e.g., all teachers within one school district) or if response rates are expected to be low. The **study population** is the group from which you select your sample. The **sampling frame** is the list of all elements that guides your sample selection from the sample population. Figure 5.1 depicts an example of the sampling process. In this example, the population is all certified school health teachers in California public elementary schools. The study population is all teachers certified to teach elementary school health education in the 200 largest school districts in California. The sampling frame is a list of certified elementary school teachers with current certification to teach elementary school health. Each individual teacher certified in elementary school health education selected from the sampling frame is an element.

Sample Size

How large of a sample do you need to answer your research questions and achieve study objectives? Having a larger sample typically reduces the risk of sampling error, but there are other considerations. What size sample is feasible to access and is within my research budget? Balancing the benefits with cost is imperative. The cost of lists, survey or intervention administration, incentives, and so on can impact the extent of the sample. (More about

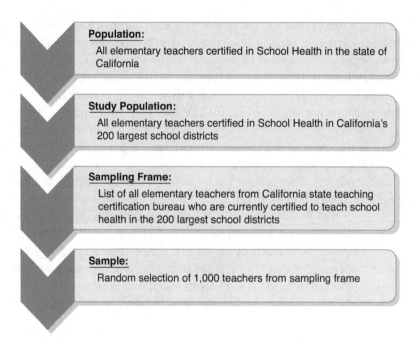

FIGURE 5.1 **The sampling process.**

research budgets is presented in Chapter 8, Developing Budgets and Timelines for Research Studies.) Choosing the best size for your sample can be tricky because a "large" sample size is relative. A sample of 100 in a small, homogenous population may be appropriate but a sample of 500 in a large, heterogeneous population would be considered too small. Adequate sample size also depends on the extent of variation within the population you study. The more homogenous the population, the more confident we can be that the sample is representative. Another consideration is the type of analyses you plan to conduct with the data. If you aim to compare two groups, such as smokers and nonsmokers, you will have to make sure enough people are in each group to make comparisons. If you want to analyze differences within these two groups by gender, you will have to make sure you have enough men and women in both the smoker and nonsmoker categories. Some statistical analyses require a minimum number in each group for valid calculations. (More about this issue is found in Chapter 10, Quantitative Data Analysis.) If you predict subgroups or subcategories will be less likely to respond or provide data, you may have to oversample in those categories. Knowing from past studies that people over 65 will be less likely to participate in your survey, and age group comparisons are vital to your research objective, you may have to include more people over 65 than the rest of the population in your sample to ensure you will have enough data.

A common method used to determine adequate sample size for public health research studies is to use statistical power calculations.[2] Power calculations determine the sample size needed to identify treatment effects or attribute differences to study interventions or treatments with a particular level of confidence. Power can be defined as the probability of rejecting the null hypothesis when it should be rejected. Federal grants as well as most institutional review boards require justification of sample size using statistical power calculations. In order to calculate sample size using power calculations, you will need some background information on the topic you wish to study, such as effect size. Effect size is the

You can learn something about sample size from M&Ms. The manufacturer, Mars Wrigley Confectionary, produces different on average percentages of each of the six colors: on average 24% blue, 20% orange, 16% green, 14% yellow, and 13% of both red and brown.[3] If you open a small bag of M&Ms and calculate the percentage of candy of each color, it will probably not match the percentages produced by the company. You are more likely to get closer to the actual percentages as you sample increasingly larger bags. The larger the sample, the more representative it is of the known population. Count freely, but consume in moderation!

quantification of differences between two or more groups. For example, from past research, you can estimate a 10% difference in weight loss between a control group and an intervention group. This effect size, predicted standard deviation of weight loss, and acceptable level of probability for random effect can be used to calculate the sample size required to accept the outcome of your hypothesis testing in your nutrition intervention study. You can use statistical software or online programs to compute sample size and power. If power calculation results show you need a minimum of 150 people in your intervention and 150 people in your control group for 80% power, this could be interpreted as the minimum number needed so that the probability of a random effect is only 20%. The higher the power, the more confident we can be in our outcomes. There is not absolute consensus on the acceptable power limits, but typically, 80% or above is adequate for most studies.[2]

SAMPLING METHODS

Characteristics of samples determine the likelihood of representing the population from which they are selected. These characteristics are based on the type of sampling methods used. There are two broad categories of sampling methods: probability and nonprobability. **Probability sampling** is used to estimate the extent to which the sample represents the larger population. Random selection is the hallmark of probability sampling. Random selection means each element within a population has an equal chance of selection, independent of any other selection. Simply stated, nothing other than chance determines which elements are included in the sample. A toss of a coin is an example of random selection. The outcome of each toss (heads or tails) is not influenced by previous tosses. The chance of the coin coming up "heads" is always 50% no matter how many times you toss the coin. This is a basic example because there are only two sides of a coin. It's not quite so simple when randomizing a larger number of people, places, or things. There are four main categories of probability sampling methods.

Simple Random Sampling. Simple random sampling occurs when elements are selected similar to a coin toss and nothing but chance influences the selection. A common method for simple random selection is to use a random numbers table. These tables are available in books and via online random number generators. Part of a random table of numbers is shown in Table 5.1. Suppose you would like to randomly select a sample of 10 similar-sized cities (from a list of 100) to include in your study. The steps needed to use a table like the one shown in Table 5.1 to randomly select your sample would be:

TABLE 5.1 EXAMPLE OF PART OF A RANDOM NUMBERS TABLE

58104	25625	19509	88916	85030
10480	81467	36207	91291	98376
30995	07856	01261	27756	96872
18876	17435	70997	49663	36320
52810	30015	11511	97735	49442
01188	71585	23495	51851	60672
15053	60045	12566	07983	31595

1. Number each city from 1 to 100.
2. Select a number from the table to begin (use Table 5.1).
3. From the starting point, go through the list in the direction of your choice to look for numbers (or the first three digits of numbers) that match your list of city numbers. If you start at the first number of the last column (85030), you can interpret it as 850, which is not on your list so move on.
4. In this example, we will move backwards. The next number at the bottom of the second-to-last column is 079. You would refer to your list and choose the city identified as number 79. Go through the list until you reach another number existing in your city list. The next relevant number would be 012, so you would select the city identified as 12.
5. Continue going through the list until you achieve your sample total.

Simple random sampling can be conducted with or without replacements. In replacement, in the number of choices for selection remains constant. If I want to randomly choose 10 numbers from a list of 100, by removing that number, the odds change from 1 in 100 to 1/99, and decrease with every subsequent choice (1/98, 1/97, 1/96). Replacement techniques keep the original selected numbers in the list or replace them with a new ones so the denominator stays consistent. As stated previously, your research purpose should drive your decisions about types of sampling method, including whether to use replacement strategies.

Systematic Random Sampling. Systematic random sampling takes simple random sampling one step further. In this method, a starting point is chosen, and then every Nth element is chosen thereafter. If you have a list of 1,000 people (in no particular order) and need a sample of 100, you could use a sampling interval of 10. You would select every 10th person on the list. This does not work for items ordered in a certain way such as an alphabetical list of last names. There are some letters that are more likely to appear as the first letter of last names than others, thus skewing the random selection. See Exhibit 5.1 for a depiction of a systematic random sample.

EXHIBIT 5.1 DEPICTION OF A SYSTEMATIC RANDOM SAMPLE

If you need a sample of 20 popular press articles on preventing osteoporosis from a list of 100 you extracted from an online search, number each of the articles, and then select every fifth one to achieve the desired sample number. The highlighted cells show which articles would be selected in this example.

1	2	3	4	5	6	7	8
9	10	11	12	13	14	15	16
17	18	19	20	21	22	23	24
25	26	27	28	29	30	31	32
33	24	35	36	37	38	39	40
41	42	43	44	45	46	47	48
49	50	51	52	53	54	55	56
57	58	59	60	61	62	63	64
65	66	67	68	69	70	71	72
73	74	75	76	77	78	79	80
81	82	83	84	85	86	87	88
89	90	91	92	93	94	95	96
97	98	99	100				

Stratified Random Sampling. Stratified random sampling is a way to draw a sample to accurately reflect a population by some defined characteristic. If you want to select a sample of 100 people from a population within a community made up of four different neighborhoods, you might stratify the sample by neighborhood, to get an equal number from each neighborhood. If you conducted a simple random sample and all 100 people were from one neighborhood, results may be less likely to represent the four neighborhoods of interest. Stratified random sampling can also be done in proportion to a particular characteristic, for example, size of neighborhood. This is called *proportionate stratified random sampling*. Of the four neighborhoods in the previous example, one has 1,000 residents, two have 2,000 residents, and one has 5,000 residents. In order to get a sample proportionate to the size of the neighborhood, you would vary (stratify) your sample number by neighborhoods. With the goal of selecting 100 people, you would select 50% of your sample from the larger neighborhood ($n = 50$) because half of the total population lives in that neighborhood. You would also select 10% ($n = 10$) from the neighborhood with 1,000 residents and 20 from each of the two neighborhoods with 2,000 people, for example. Stratified random sampling is often used in public health research to match the sample to the demographics of a given population. Race/ethnicity, gender, and education level are common factors on which to base stratification. The U.S. Census provides data for many demographic characteristics from which you can base your stratified sample.

Cluster Random Sampling. Cluster random sampling is similar to stratified random sampling, in that groups are the primary selection. This may occur in a single step or in multiple stages. In a multistage cluster sample, the groups are selected first, and then elements are randomly selected within those groups. For a study of students, you might randomly select school districts using stratified random or another random selection technique, and then from the districts selected, randomly choose teachers within those districts to survey for your study. The district is the "cluster" from which the final sample of elements is selected. It is much easier to find a list of all U.S. school districts than a list of all U.S. schoolteachers. You can do a multistage cluster sampling with three levels if it is relevant to your research objective. Geographic regions, such as counties, can be selected in the first stage. Within each randomly selected county, you could then randomly choose zip codes. From those zip codes, you could randomly choose individual residents to serve as your sample. It is important to note, however, that cluster sampling has a higher risk of sampling error than simple random sampling does. Sampling error increases as the number of selected clusters decrease. The fewer the clusters selected, the higher the sampling error due to potential homogeneity within each cluster.

RANDOM DIGIT DIALING

Random-digit dialing was once a staple of data collection. In this method, the area code or the first three numbers and the prefix (the next three numbers) are randomly selected. With these six numbers kept constant, the final four numbers are randomly selected. Calls are made to the completed sequence of telephone numbers. For example, if (314) 271was the sequence selected, the list of possible combinations of the last four numbers would be randomly generated and added (e.g., 314-271-1234, 314-271-4567, etc.). The area codes and prefixes are known as *clusters*. Landline phone numbers have area codes linked to geographic area. If homogeneity exists within area codes/geographic regions, the risk of sampling error increases. With the change in telephone culture, people are using mobile phones instead of landlines, and phone numbers may not be linked to current geographic region. This increases heterogeneity in the selected area code prefix combination, making the risk of sampling error lower than it is in landline number clusters. Now if people would only answer their phones!

The second broad category of sampling method is **nonprobability,** or nonrandom sampling. In public health research, there are many situations in which it is not possible or feasible to use a random sample. A complete sample frame may not exist, so individuals may not have an equal and independent chance of being selected. Because of this, you cannot estimate the effect of sampling error, which may reduce representativeness and generalizability to the larger population. In spite of this limitation of nonprobability sampling, there are benefits to using this method. Although you may not be able to precisely determine error and representativeness, convenience and lower cost make this method common in public health research. However, a key consideration is sample quality. Researchers need to ensure adequate sample size and implement the sampling plan using best practices. Detailed reporting of sampling procedures is also needed. Remember, evidence is built on research. Studies using similar sampling techniques among different populations can build the evidence for the effectiveness of public health programs, policies, and interventions. There are four main categories of nonprobability sampling methods.

Convenience sampling. A convenience (or availability) sampling method takes advantage of easy-to-access people, places, or things to study (Figure 5.2). Has someone collecting survey data ever approached you in a public space? This person is using anyone who walks by as their "convenience" sample. Asking for volunteers to participate in a research study is also a way of gathering a convenience sample. Convenience samples are especially relevant for student research assignments. If you want to explore attitudes on gun violence research among public health students, it would be easy to gain access to your classmates or other people in your cohort.

Purposive sampling. The purposive (or criterion) sampling method is based on some prior knowledge about the sample population. Based on your research aims, you set criteria for inclusion or exclusion of whom you want to participate or places/things you want in your study. For example, if you want to survey state legislators on their perceptions of obesity-prevention policies, they need to have some knowledge of the topic in order to provide useful insight. A target criterion for inclusion in your sample might be membership on the legislative health committee. Targeting specific subsets of the population based on characteristics meaningful to the research purpose can be an efficient way to gather data.

Quota sampling. Quota sampling means setting proportional goals based on sample characteristics. This method is a way to demonstrate representativeness of those characteristics to the larger population. Suppose you want to explore perceptions of stress in graduate students at your university. You hypothesize this perception may vary by discipline. You know the number of students in each graduate school varies greatly, so you use this information to develop a quota-sampling method. Quota sampling is like a nonrandom stratified

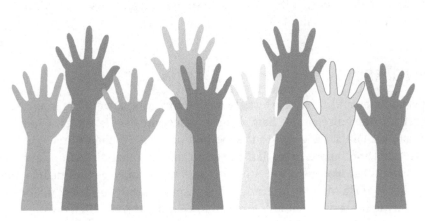

FIGURE 5.2 **Convenience sample.**

TABLE 5.2 QUOTA SAMPLING			
Graduate School	Number of Students	Percentage of All Graduate Students	Number Needed for Quota Sampling for $N = 200$
Medicine	300	30	60
Law	160	16	32
Public health	210	21	42
Business	200	20	40
Engineering	130	13	26
	1,000	100	200

method. Even though you are not using random selection, you can sample in a way that represents the characteristic of interest (e.g., size of each graduate school). See Table 5.2 for an example.

Snowball sampling. Just as a snowball grows as it rolls down a snowy hill, a snowball sample gets larger as the research project advances. In snowball sampling, you identify a small number of participants and, during data collection, and ask them to identify others who are relevant to your study. This method is useful for populations that may be harder to reach or less likely to respond. Snowball sampling capitalizes on established relationships or connectively within groups. If you want to explore how parents within a certain school perceive new lunch criteria, you can gain access to a larger group by starting with a few key people. Identify the formal or informal leaders within the population of interest for the start of your snowball sample. They will likely be able to provide others to participate in your study. This method is used frequently in exploratory or qualitative studies. Consider the sensitivity of your research topic when selecting this method. Some people may not want to be identified by other study participants. Privacy, societal perceptions, and cultural norms are ethical criteria for snowball sampling.

SAMPLING ISSUES

Sampling is complex and rarely perfect. Two common issues, sampling bias and sampling error, warrant further discussion. **Sampling or selection bias** is the misrepresentation of some population characteristic due to the method of selecting the sample. Bias may be the result of several factors, and is more likely to occur in nonprobability samples than ones that are randomly selected. For instance, suppose you conduct a survey of people entering the community library on a Monday afternoon. The responses only represent (a) those who visit the library during the day, potentially underrepresenting those with daytime employment;

(b) people who visit the library, potentially underrepresenting people who read books or online resources; and/or (c) adults who are not in school, potentially underrepresenting school-aged adolescents or young adults. These are all contributors to sampling bias.

Self-selection can also result in bias. Perhaps the only people to volunteer for a weight-loss study will be those already motivated to lose weight. In addition, sampling bias can occur when some members of the intended population are less likely to be included than the general population. For example, an online survey eliminates the input from anyone who does not have Internet access. Equity is an important consideration when developing your sampling plan. Snowball sampling may result in bias, too. If you ask people for referrals to other participants, they may recommend like-minded people. There may be less variation in your snowball sample than a sample derived from other methods. In order to reduce sampling bias use random methods if possible. This "equal opportunity" method reduces bias selection. If random methods are not a viable option, define the sampling frame so that it is as representative as possible to the larger population.

Nonresponse bias may occur when you do not reach all members in your sample. Replacing cases with inaccurate contact information (e.g., email bounce backs or returned mail surveys) is a way to improve your sample. Nonresponse bias may also be due to differences in characteristics of those who respond and those who do not. Imagine a survey on the perceptions of clean indoor air policies. Certain factors (e.g., smoking status) may influence whether a person responds. The findings will not accurately represent the views of the general population (smokers and nonsmokers) due to nonresponse bias. Oversampling or providing incentives may increase response rates. Monitor the characteristics of the respondents for consistency with the target population to mitigate nonresponse bias if needed.

The result of sampling bias is **sampling error.** Sample estimates of population parameters are often incorrect. *Sampling error* is defined as the difference between the results from a sample population when compared to results from the whole population. The most common outcome of sampling error is systematic error. As mentioned in Chapter 4, Operationalization and Measurement, systematic error is due to flaws in measurement and reduces the strength of research results. There are recommendations for reducing sampling error such as increasing sample size and using random selection.

Random selection also allows for calculating inferential statistics. These procedures use statistical models to compare sample data to population data or samples from other research studies. Inferential statistics are discussed in greater detail in Chapter 10, Quantitative Data Analysis. If using random selection or increasing sample size are not feasible options, look to past studies for ways to implement the most rigorous sampling methods for your research objectives.

An important aspect of assessing research quality is to scrutinize who or what makes up the sample. When reading published research studies or even popular press coverage of public health research, ask these three questions:
- **From what population were cases selected?**
- **What method was used to select cases from this population?**
- **Do the cases represent the population from which they were selected?**

CHAPTER DISCUSSION QUESTIONS

1. Describe two ways you might develop a sample for a study to answer the research question: "Do text-message reminders work to increase flu vaccine uptake in low-wage hospital employees?" Discuss the advantages and disadvantages of both methods.
2. What are some ramifications of nonresponse bias for underrepresented groups in research?
3. Weigh the pros and cons of large samples versus small samples for studies with limited funding.
4. Identify two ways you could use cluster stratified sampling to design a sample for a study on community access to baby-friendly hospitals.

RESEARCH PROJECT CHECK-IN

Who, What, and How?

It doesn't matter if you plan to study people, places, documents, or other phenomenon—you need a sampling plan. Use the information in this chapter to develop the best ways to sample for your study. Because this is a class project, there may be limitations in sampling method due to feasibility. Think beyond the course-required study parameters. If you were conducting this as a real-world research study, how would you sample? Give careful consideration to the ethics of sampling, too. "Unplanned selectiveness" can be a detriment to study rigor and generalizability.

PUBLIC HEALTH RESEARCH METHODS IN REAL LIFE

A Tale of Two Samples

Six months ago, a statewide campaign to "FILL UP ON FRESH" was implemented to encourage consumption of fresh fruits and vegetables. Nadja represented the state health department on a collaborative team in charge of development, implementation, and evaluation of the project. One aspect of the campaign was a partnership with grocery stores throughout the state to provide them with promotional materials for use in their produce department. The team developed a complex evaluation plan to measure program effectiveness. Nadja was in charge of part of the evaluation intended to determine the extent to which stores posted the promotional materials in their produce section and provided customers with "FILL UP ON FRESH" bags. Her first task with this assignment was to develop a sample.

They did not have the time or resources to go to all 997 stores in the state. Several people on the research team recommended a random sample in order to get the most representative and generalizable group of stores to evaluate. Nadja remembered from her public health research methods class that the concept of randomness means every unit has an equal chance of being selected for the sample. She already had a list of all stores in the state. Of the 997 stores on this list, they were aiming for about 185 (20%) stores to evaluate. She decided to use a table of random numbers to help her select the stores. The list of stores contained a three-digit grocer ID number that was assigned by the state grocery store trade association. Nadja would use the ID number to match to the random numbers table. She selected 185 stores using this method.

She brought the list of stores to the research team at the next evaluation meeting. She also brought a map of the randomly selected stores. Once mapped, she noticed that most of the stores were located in one region (bordering the adjacent state). She wanted to consider any potential regional variations when interpreting data on whether stores used promotional products provided by the "FILL UP ON FRESH" program. The research team agreed and asked her to come up with another sample that was distributed throughout the state.

Nadja decided a stratified sample might be a better strategy to use for her evaluation task. The state is divided into six geographic regions used by many state agencies for resource distribution. Each of these geographic regions would be a strata for the sample. Each strata contained about the same number grocery stores. She went back to the list of stores and divided them by region. Nadja randomly selected 31 stores from each of the six regions for a total sample of 186 stores to evaluate. The research team supported this new sample and was eager to start evaluating the implementation of the campaign.

Critical Thinking Questions

1. Why do you think a random sample was chosen over other methods? What are the benefits of random selection for this campaign evaluation?
2. What other ways could Nadja have selected a random sample of stores?
3. What would be the challenge of evaluating every single store in the state? What are the benefits and disadvantages of using the full list?
4. How might her first sample of stores impact evaluation results?
5. What are other ways to stratify the stores in the state?

COUNCIL ON EDUCATION FOR PUBLIC HEALTH FOUNDATIONAL KNOWLEDGE AND COMPETENCIES

Foundational Knowledge

Profession and Science of Public Health

- Explain the critical importance of evidence in advancing public health knowledge.

Foundational Competencies

Evidence-Based Approaches to Public Health

- Select quantitative and qualitative data-collection methods appropriate for a given public health context.

Planning and Management to Promote Health

- Assess population needs, assets, and capabilities that affect communities' health.
- Select methods to evaluate public health programs.

REFERENCES

1. Woolsey TD, Cochran WG, Mainland D, Martin MP, Moore Jr FE, Patton RE. On the use of sampling in the field of public health. *Am J Public Health*. 1954;44(6):720–740. doi:10.2105/AJPH.44.6.719

2. Cohen J. *Statistical Power Analysis for the Behavioral Sciences*. 2nd ed. New York, NY: Lawrence Erlbaum Associates; 1988.

3. Wicklin R. The distribution of colors for plain M&M candies. SAS Blogs. February 20, 2017. Accessed September 3, 2020. https://blogs.sas.com/content/iml/2017/02/20/proportion-of-colors-mandms.html

ADDITIONAL READINGS AND RESOURCES

Bacchetti P, Wolff LE, Seagl MR, et al. Ethics and sample size. *Am J Epidemiol*. 2005;161(2):105–110. https://academic.oup.com/aje/article/161/2/105/256528

Lwanga SK, Lemeshow S. *Sample Size Determination in Health Studies: A Practical Manual*. Geneva, Switzerland: World Health Organization; 1991. https://apps.who.int/iris/handle/10665/40062

Random.org. Random integer generator. n.d. Accessed August 15, 2019. https://www.random.org/integers

6

Quantitative Study Designs: Experimental

Correlation is not causation.

—Karl Pearson, mathematician

INTRODUCTION

There are many ways to study a public health issue. Consider the topic of electric cigarettes or vaping. You could explore the facilitators of vaping among adolescents, describe the correlates of use, explain the determinants of use, or evaluate the effectiveness of a program or policy to reduce this behavior. As stated in Chapter 1, The Importance of Research in Public Health, the main purpose of research (exploration, description, explanation, and evaluation) informs the ways a study is planned and implemented. The purpose drives study design. For example, explorative and descriptive studies typically do not rely on proving cause and effect. However, if the research purpose is to explain or fully evaluate the effectiveness of a program or policy, certain study design requirements have to be met. Suppose your research question is "Does the tailored stress-management intervention improve sleep health in adults?" You use probability sampling to identify a sample of 100 people already enrolled in a large stress-management program. You randomly assign 50 of them to get a tailored sleep health intervention as part of stress management. The other 50 people get the usual intervention. If the intervention group reports better sleep duration and quality compared to the usual care group, we would be able to infer the tailored sleep health intervention was the reason for the difference. In this simplified description of the sleep health study, we need to determine that it was, in fact, the intervention and nothing else that contributed to the difference between groups in the outcome measure. The type of study design influences the level of certainty in making this inference.

In order to conclude the independent variable (intervention) caused the change to our dependent variable (sleep duration and quality), the three criteria for causal inference must be met. Although with some variation, there is a fair amount of consensus in the scientific community for three criteria used for causal inference in general research. The first criterion for inferring causality is **association**. The independent and dependent variables must covary with one another or be associated in some way. A change in one will result in a change in the other. Without an association, there can be no causal relationship. The second criterion for inferring causality is order in time. **The cause must precede the effect.** This may seem obvious, but it needs to be validated. Suppose you find that most people who washed their hands throughout the day watched a popular movie about a deadly flu outbreak and most people who reported not washing their hands throughout the day did not watch the movie. You think there is an association between handwashing and the movie, only to find out the handwashing data was collected before the movie was released. Because the dependent variable (handwashing) occurred before the independent variable (the movie), we cannot infer that watching the movie caused the difference in handwashing behavior. The third criterion for inferring causality is **nonspuriousness**. This means the covariation between the two variables cannot be explained as the result of influence of some other variable. The association between two variables might be caused by something else. We need to design our studies in a way to ensure the only influence on the dependent variable is the independent variable and the variation is not due to a third (i.e., extraneous) variable.

To recap, the three criteria for inferring causality are

1. the variables must be associated or covary,
2. the cause must precede the effect in time, and
3. the relationship cannot be explained by a third variable of influence.

INTERNAL VALIDITY

Chapter 4, Operationalization and Measurement, describes internal validity as the extent to which a measure accurately depicts what it is intended to measure. Related to causal inference, internal validity means the study results accurately represent causation. This concept refers to the confidence that the three criteria for inferring causality are met. In an internally valid study, you are sure the two variables are associated, are in the correct time order, and no third variable contributed to the association. Some aspects of a study can interfere with internal validity. There are several threats to internal validity common in public health research. Careful study design, implementation, and data analysis can reduce the risk and impact of these threats.

Selection Bias

Chapter 5, Sampling, defines sampling bias, or creating a sample that is not representative due to a variety of factors. Selection bias is different. Although sample bias means the sample may be different from the target population, this type of bias occurs when the groups in your study are not comparable. In the previous sleep health intervention example, what if you asked for volunteers to participate in the intervention and put all those who refused into the control group? We cannot be certain the improvement in sleep duration and quality in the intervention group was not due to characteristics of people in each group. The groups were not comparable. Random assignment into the intervention and control groups is one way to reduce selection bias. In many public health research studies, however, random assignment may not be feasible or ethical. Imagine studying the impact of some environmental change. One community in the study area is exposed to the change, while the other is not. You cannot randomly place residents into communities to fit your study design. In this example the criteria for inferring causality are not met, and because of nonrandom assignment, a third variable (e.g., participant characteristic) might influence the outcome. Causality is an important outcome of research, but it is not the only reason to conduct studies. There still is value in findings from studies that do not meet the criteria for causality. Quasi-experimental studies, as discussed in Chapter 7, Quantitative Study Designs: Nonexperimental, make valid contributions to public health evidence.

History

This bias does not refer to things you might have learned in high school history class. Events occurring during the course of your research study can impact the outcome. Suppose you implement a distracted-driving awareness intervention in a community. During the intervention, one of the town's elected officials is involved in a crash caused by texting while driving. The story is published in all of the local news outlets. The change in awareness of the risks of distracted driving may not have been solely due to your intervention. People may have been made more aware of the issue from the news story. Although you do not have control over such extraneous events, they need to be reported as a limitation when you write up the study results.

In 1998, the husband of well-known news celebrity Katie Couric died of colon cancer. He was 42. Ms. Couric was devastated by his death and became a fierce advocate for awareness of this disease. In March 2000, she underwent a live on-air colonoscopy on the *Today Show* as part of a weeklong focus on colon cancer awareness and the importance of colon cancer screening. The result was a temporary increase in colonoscopy use. Dubbed the "Katie Couric effect," research findings on this topic suggest a celebrity spokesperson can have a substantial impact on public participation in preventive-care programs. This also poses an example of how extraneous events can impact research outcomes. The death of her husband and Ms. Couric's advocacy could have been a threat to internal validity of any other colon cancer intervention going on at the same time.[11]

Testing

Testing can contribute to improved performance in and of itself. Think about how much time and effort some high school students put into practicing for the American College Testing (ACT) or Scholastic Assessment Test (SAT) exams. They take the tests over and over to increase their scores. Their knowledge of the subjects may not increase, but their test-taking skills improve. Sometimes in research, the process of testing or assessment creates improvement, not necessarily due to improvements in the construct it is measuring. This may result in failure to find any significant intervention effects because both intervention and control groups achieved better outcomes due to testing effects. Assessments can act as an intervention. Suppose you design a weight-loss study with randomly selected intervention and control groups. Weighing the control group participants at baseline might incite behaviors conducive to weight loss, even if they are not exposed to the intervention. Certain study designs can be implemented to rule out testing effects.

Maturation

Research studies are implemented over time, and the effect of time may produce short- or long-term changes in the participants of your study. These changes can impact your results. Short-term maturation effects may be due to changes in mood of the participant because of tiredness or boredom. Although a researcher may not be able to control how much sleep a participant gets before the intervention occurs, they can try to reduce participant burden and consider potential short-term maturation effects in study design. Long-term maturation changes include aging, advancing in education, or increasing/decreasing income. These changes can occur within time frames of a few months to years. Think about how much growth and development happens during puberty. A long-term study on food intake and weight on young adolescents would definitely have to consider the potential effects of maturation. Employment, childbirth, and retirement can contribute to maturation effects in adults. Older adults may experience physical or cognitive changes during the time period of a study. Reviewing the literature and fully exploring your research topic will help determine the potential extent of maturation as a threat to internal validity.

Attrition

If participants drop out before study completion, this may affect study outcome. In longer term health studies, mortality may reduce the study sample at posttest. Attrition can be a threat to internal validity when those who drop out are significantly different from participants remaining in the study. For example, in a 12-week intervention to prevent cardiovascular disease, 40% of participants drop out after week 6. Upon inquiry, you find out most of those who dropped out were laid off from their jobs at a local employer when a factory shut down. The characteristic (employment) between those who remained in class versus those who dropped out can be a significant limitation to study findings. At the end of your study, you can statistically compare characteristics of those who dropped out with those who remained in the study in order to identify attrition bias. High attrition may also cause analysis difficulties, especially if you need a minimum group number to determine statistical significance. As a preventive measure, make sure the sample is large enough to accommodate potential attrition. Information from past studies may provide helpful information about attrition in specific population groups.

There are several ways to reduce the potential for attrition bias. The use of incentives, or providing some type of compensation, is one strategy recommended to maintain participation in research studies. Graduated incentives may be effective in keeping people involved in longer term studies. With this method, participants are offered a choice of smaller incentives (typically monetary) at each intervention segment, or a larger incentive to be received at the end of the study. For example, in a 6-month evaluation of the impact of a campaign to reduce sugar-sweetened beverage intake among high school students, students might be offered $10 after completing the baseline survey, $10 at the 3-month survey, and 10$ at the 6-month follow-up. The other incentive option might be to provide $50 to each participant who completes the third survey at 6 months (versus a total of $30 if they take the incentive in increments). Another strategy to reduce attrition is through follow-up with participants. You will need accurate contact information as well as preferred method of contact for effective follow-up, as well as dedicated research staff time for comprehensive follow-up.

Statistical Regression

Statistical regression as a threat to internal validity has to do with "room for improvement." When scores from assessment are particularly high or low, there is a tendency for these scores to move toward the mean or average score. Let's use physical activity as an example. People who are mostly sedentary (i.e., take less than 1,000 steps per day) will likely show improvement in a walking intervention because they have such low activity to begin with. If more sedentary people are in the intervention group, they will show greater improvement. Researchers can reduce the risk of statistical regression as a threat to internal validity by using random group assignment and reliable measures.

Instrumentation Changes

Internal validity may be compromised if the instrument or measuring device changes over time. These changes can be due to the researcher or the actual measuring device. For example, at the beginning of an intervention your study team takes photos to analyze outdoor smoking spaces. At the end of the intervention, your team conducts observations of the same spaces. There may be differences in the factors captured by these two methods. Consistency in the measuring instrument is important. Both photos and observations can be valid ways to assess the spaces, but may not be comparable. In addition, changes may happen to the measurement device over the course of the study. Suppose you use a tape measure to calculate the amount of space allotted to tobacco products in grocery stores. After the 25th store, the tape measure becomes stretched out. The measurements taken at the stores at the beginning might be slightly different from those measured later in the study. Study design should include consistent and precise measures.

THE HAWTHORNE EFFECT

Just knowing research is being conducted may result in a change in study participants' behavior. This phenomenon is termed the *Hawthorne effect* after productivity experiments conducted between 1924 and 1932 at Hawthorne Works, a factory outside of Chicago, Illinois. Company leaders wanted to study how levels of light in the workspaces influenced productivity. The workers' productivity increased in both high and low lighting but decreased when the study concluded. Other studies at Hawthorne showed similar change patterns, where improvements existed until the study ended. The workers seemed to be motivated by the studies, not necessarily the environmental changes that were part of the intervention. In 1958, Henry A. Landsberger, a sociologist who studied industrial and labor relations, analyzed the data from the Hawthorne studies and coined the term *Hawthorne effect* to mean short-lived increases in productivity. Even though this phenomenon has been studied for over seven decades, there is a need for empirical studies to identify the magnitude, conditions, and mechanisms of the Hawthorne effect.[12]

Compensatory Rivalry

This threat to internal validity occurs in studies using more than one group. Participants aware of the group design may become competitive. Those in the control group, for example, might improve in the outcome measure even though they were not exposed to the intervention due to rivalry with the other group. This is sometimes called the John Henry effect. John Henry is a folk-tale hero. In the story, he was a strong, African American railroad worker. When he became aware his work was being compared to that of a steam drill, he put forth so much extra effort that the added exertion killed him.[1] Compensatory rivalry in research studies is not just folklore. Consider a worksite wellness intervention to facilitate weight loss. Participants in the control group may work harder to lose weight due to competition with their coworkers, who are assigned to the intervention group. Getting input from the sample population during planning can help the research team develop strategies to minimize the potential for this threat to internal validity.

Compensatory Demoralization

When people are assigned to the control group instead of the intervention group, they may feel resentful or disadvantaged. This, in turn, may affect their commitment to the study and the level of differences in outcome between the groups. Dropout rates may also increase in participants with feelings of compensatory demoralization. Imagine a study on cognitive benefits of exercise in older adults. One group gets private sessions with a personal trainer while they work out on an exercise bicycle and one group follows a self-guided series of stretches. The room in which they complete the stretching has a big glass window into the area of the exercise bicycles. The stretching group can see the bicycle group having fun, while they lie on the floor and stretch. The stretching group feels demoralized for not being chosen for the intervention group. Even if all participants get a free gym membership after the study ends, those in the stretching group may become less engaged and more likely to drop out of the study.

THE PLACEBO EFFECT

Placebos are treatments that have no effect (e.g., sugar pill), but that are given to participants to make them think they are being treated. A placebo effect occurs when participants receiving a placebo show improvement in the outcome compared with participants who receive no treatment (i.e., no placebo or intervention). Psychological outcomes, such as perceived effort or pain tolerance, are more vulnerable to placebo effects than physiological outcomes. "Blinding" is sometimes used in placebo studies. In blinded studies, participants do not know whether they are receiving the treatment or the placebo until the study ends. In double-blinded studies, both the researchers and the participants do not know who is receiving the treatment and who is receiving the placebo. The use of a placebo control group can also be a way to differentiate the impact of placebo effect on internal validity. If the risk for placebo effect is high, a researcher would design a study with three groups: an intervention group (receiving treatment), a placebo group (receiving a placebo), and a control group (receiving no treatment or placebo). The use of placebos is more common in medical research than in public health research. However, the concept of "the placebo" can be integrated into public health studies in some cases. Crum and Langer[2] conducted a study on the health of 84 female hotel cleaners. They told half of the participants that the work they did counted as exercise and they were active enough to achieve the recommended amounts of physical activity as per the U.S. physical activity guidelines. The other half of the participants were provided with no information other than they were participating in a health study. Although their behavior did not change during the 4-week intervention, the informed group perceived themselves as getting more exercise than at baseline. They also showed improvements in weight, body mass index, blood pressure, and waist-to-hip ratio.[2] We know from Chapter 1, The Importance of Research in Public Health, that one small study does not provide conclusive evidence on the efficacy of placebo effect on exercise, but it is a unique, nonmedical example of a placebo study.

EXPERIMENTAL STUDY DESIGNS

The features within study designs define the extent to which we can determine whether the change in our outcome of interest (dependent variable) was due to our independent variable. **Experimental study designs** have features providing the highest level of control for threats to internal validity, while meeting the three criteria for inferring causality. In experimental studies, participants are randomly assigned to either an experimental group or a control group. Each group is assessed, the experimental group receives the intervention or treatment, and both groups are reassessed. The results of the outcome of interest are compared between the two groups. The classic experimental study design is the **pretest–posttest control group design**. This design can be drawn as follows:

$$\begin{array}{cccc} R & O_1 & X & O_2 \\ R & O_1 & & O_2 \end{array}$$

In this depiction, **R** stands for random assignment into intervention or control groups, which is a hallmark of the experimental design. O_1 stands for pretest or baseline measures. The **X** is the intervention or treatment (not given to control group). O_2 stands for posttest. These notations are commonly used to outline study designs. The pretest–posttest study design is also shown in Exhibit 6.1.

This design has features to control for threats to internal validity. Look at the study example in Exhibit 6.1. Selection bias is reduced or eliminated through random group assignment. The groups of adolescents should be comparable. Random selection also makes it less likely that one group would be more likely to statistically regress from extreme score to mean scores than the other group. Any changes in stress perception due to maturation would be seen in both groups. Pretest–posttest control group design is common in public health research. See Table 6.1 for some examples. One threat to internal validity that may be a concern when using this study design is testing. A **posttest-only control group design** eliminates the impact of the testing effect. This design is similar to pretest–posttest control group design, but without the pretest. It can be depicted as:

$$\begin{array}{ccc} R & X & O \\ R & & O \end{array}$$

What if in order to answer your research question, you still need to determine differences between pre- and posttest measures, but there is the potential threat of a testing effect? You could use a **Solomon four-group study design**. This combines the classic pretest–posttest control group design with the posttest-only control group design. All groups are randomly assigned, but two get the intervention; one intervention group with pretest, and one intervention group without pretest. This design also has two control groups: one control group with

EXHIBIT 6.1 BASIC EXPERIMENTAL DESIGN: PRETEST–POSTTEST CONTROL GROUP

Experimental Group		Control Group
Pretest	-------compare------	Pretest
(Intervention)		
Posttest	-------compare------	Posttest

TABLE 6.1 EXAMPLES OF PRETEST–POSTTEST CONTROL GROUP DESIGNS IN PUBLIC HEALTH RESEARCH	
Citation	Description
Swartz et al.[3]	Randomized to intervention group of students and waitlist controls for depression literacy. Used pretest assessment and a 4-month follow-up.
Mutanski et al.[4]	HIV-negative men randomly assigned to eHealth intervention or control condition. Baseline assessment and postdata collected 3, 6, and 12 months after intervention.
Garrison et al.[5]	Participants assigned to intervention or usual experience and measured smoking abstinence 1 week and 6 months postintervention.
Crosby et al.[6]	Participants were randomized to interactive intervention or attention-equivalent control condition. Assessments occurred at baseline, 2, and 6 months after intervention.
Connor et al.[7]	Women aged 18 to 25 were randomly assigned to 14-day intervention or diet-as-usual conditions. Depression and anxiety were measured pre- and postintervention.
Chang et al.[8]	Participants randomized to community health worker intervention or usual care. Pretest measures and posttest performed on access and utilization after 1 year.

pretest, and one control group without pretest. If testing influences change the outcome, you would find differences when comparing the experimental groups with each other as well as comparing the results between the two control groups. The Solomon four-group design can be drawn as:

$$
\begin{array}{cccc}
R & O_1 & X & O_2 \\
R & O_1 & & O_2 \\
R & & X & O_2 \\
R & & & O_2 \\
\end{array}
$$

Suppose you are interested in the effects of an intervention to increase safe-sex practices among college students. The intervention consists of a 2-hour peer-led information session on sexual health. You want to get a baseline assessment of knowledge about sexual health and safe-sex practices, but past literature indicates high risk for testing effects in this type of study. During student orientation, you randomly assign students to four groups and provide the intervention to two of the four groups. You conduct a pretest in two groups (one experimental and one control) and, after 30 days, collect posttest data from participants in all four groups. Your analysis of group results shows significant differences in safe-sex practices among the groups with and without the pretest. You conclude that it was not the intervention, but the pretest, that influenced changes in safe-sex practices.

Public health interventions can be complex and multifaceted. For interventions having multiple components, researchers may be interested in studying the effectiveness of each component separately, or different combinations of components. Maybe the whole intervention is not needed to create the desired outcome. Resources can be used more judiciously if there is evidence on the most efficient ways to deliver interventions. **Dismantling study designs** look at the whole intervention, but also break down the intervention components. This type of design is depicted as:

$$R \quad O_1 \quad X_{AB} \quad O_2$$
$$R \quad O_1 \quad X_A \quad O_2$$
$$R \quad O_1 \quad X_B \quad O_2$$
$$R \quad O_1 \quad \quad O_2$$

Here, **AB** stands for the whole intervention, and both **A** and **B** separately depict separate intervention strategies or components. As in the other experimental designs, a control group gets no intervention. This type of study design is becoming increasingly important in public health research—technological advances are providing more options for intervention delivery. Let us use as an example a nutrition intervention with two components. The intervention consists of an in-person series of classes coupled with weekly online modules. With dismantling, the researcher can compare the effectiveness of the whole intervention, the in-person component and the online component.

Another experimental study design important for public health research is called the **alternative treatment design**. This design is similar to dismantling, but only separate components (not the components together) are investigated. Alternative treatment design is drawn as:

$$R \quad O_1 \quad X_A \quad O_2$$
$$R \quad O_1 \quad X_B \quad O_2$$
$$R \quad O_1 \quad \quad O_2$$

The intervention or strategies are represented by X_A and X_B. Let us say you have two feasible intervention options for fall prevention among community-dwelling older adults. X_A represents an intervention in which health educators make home visits to suggest environmental modifications to reduce risk of falling. X_B represents an intervention in which participants get the same information in a group setting at the local library. You collect data on home risk for falls at baseline and again at posttest for all three groups. You study the different interventions or "alternative treatments" separately and compare them to no intervention (control group).

The decision on which experimental design to use should be based on several factors. These questions may help you decide:

- What is the purpose of my research?
- Which design will provide results to answer my research question?
- What threats to internal validity do I anticipate?
- What lessons learned or recommendations can be found in the literature about my topic of study?
- What study design is feasible and can be implemented with my available resources?

THE ETHICAL CHALLENGE OF CONTROL GROUPS

Is it ethical to withhold potentially beneficial strategies or services from participants in control groups for the sake of developing evidence? The control group is a hallmark of experimental study designs, but control group participants may be at a disadvantage if the intervention shows effectiveness. This remains an ethical issue in many public health and medical studies. For pharmaceutical studies, the U.S. Food and Drug Administration specifically outlines the types of control groups to be used and when they are appropriate.[9] There have been cases in which the experimental drug is so effective, the study is halted and control group participants get the experimental drug.[10]

It important to balance the rigor of using control groups in experimental studies with ethical research practices. Researchers may opt to use a wait-list control group (where the intervention is given to the control group after a period of time). This provides data on the treatment effects, but also allows all participants to gain potential benefits of the intervention. Institutional review boards will identify potential ethical issues with study design and require changes before study implementation. Know the research topic well before designing your study. Look to past studies for control group best practice recommendations.

CHAPTER DISCUSSION QUESTIONS

1. What factors would you consider when designing a study to answer the research question: "How effective is XYZ intervention in reducing preterm birth among low-income pregnant teens?"
2. Discuss how sample size might affect internal validity.
3. What public health research topics might not be appropriate or ethical for random assignment of study participants?
4. What could you do to reduce the threat of compensatory rivalry and compensatory demoralization?

RESEARCH PROJECT CHECK-IN

Causality, Validity, and Design

Think about the potential threats to internal validity for your proposed study. What are ways you could reduce the potential for these factors? How did past studies on similar topics or within similar populations address these threats? How might you design your study to best answer your research question or achieve the study aim? Even if you are not planning to conduct an experimental study design, it is vital to understand the parameters of causality. This knowledge will help you critically analyze findings from other studies throughout your time as a student, and well into your public health career.

PUBLIC HEALTH RESEARCH METHODS IN REAL LIFE

A Causality for Concern

If there was one thing Natalicio remembered from his public health research methods class it was "correlation is not causation." This message was repeated over and over again to get students to understand that just because things are related in some way, we cannot say *X* caused *Y* unless certain parameters were met. Natalicio was asked to look into the literature and make recommendations for designing a study. He worked for a large hospital system in the division of employee health. Employee data showed a recent spike in the prevalence of injuries among patient transport workers. His boss wanted to implement an evidence-based intervention on safe lifting and back health with the patient transport workers. Before the hospital administration would sign off on the investment in the intervention for all patient transport workers, they wanted proof that it would reduce the injury rate among this population.

Natalicio looked to the published literature on the intervention to get some ideas for the proposed study design. There were several papers published available because it was the subject of a national multisite randomized control trial. The program was implemented in three large hospital systems in three different states. Patient transport workers at each site were randomized into the intervention group (where they took part in a four-session educational program on safe lifting and back health) or a control group (where they received no education). The program resulted in a significant decrease in injuries among patient transport workers in the intervention group compared with those in the control group at all three sites. However, the articles brought up a few threats to internal validity. First, the workers in both groups worked at the same place and often socialized during breaks and before they clocked in. At one of the research sites, it was anecdotally reported that some of the workers in the control group felt as if they were disadvantaged because they were not in the group that received the training on injury prevention. Data from another site showed a decrease in the injuries among workers in the control group. The difference between the intervention and control group at that site was still statistically significant but pointed to a potential Hawthorne effect. All sites reported attrition in program attendance.

Natalicio made note of all of the information reported in the articles so he could propose a study design that used the best possible methods to account for potential threats to internal validity. He also wanted to make sure he was using an experimental design that met the criteria for causality. He designed a pretest–posttest control group study for the patient transport workers at the hospital. He thought about ways to reduce interactions with the workers in the control group. One way was to separate them by shift. The rates of injuries were similar in those who worked the morning shift compared to those who worked in the afternoon. He decided to randomly select workers on the afternoon shift to receive the intervention, and randomly select workers from the morning shift for the control group. He made sure the groups were similar in characteristics for comparability. Workers on the afternoon shift were told that everyone would eventually be required to complete the safe lifting and back health program, but administration was implementing it in smaller groups. Control group participants or any of the morning-shift workers received any communication about the program. In order to combat attrition, the program was offered during the workday as part of the normal 8-hour shift. Posttest measures would be prevalence of injuries from patient transport at 4 weeks, 12 weeks, and 6 months after the program.

Natalicio took the study-design plan to his boss for approval. Although it was not perfect, his boss felt it was rigorous enough to demonstrate the effectiveness of the intervention among patient transport workers. They could use the results to gain administration support for full-scale implementation.

Critical Thinking Questions

1. What are the advantages of duplicating an intervention that is well represented in the literature?
2. What other experimental designs would have worked with this population?
3. Contamination between the intervention and control group was reported as a potential threat. What are other ways Natalicio could have designed the two groups to reduce this contamination?
4. What if the demographics of the patient transport workers were significantly different in Natalicio's hospital compared to what was reported in the literature?
5. Was it ethical to withhold the intervention to the control group if evidence showed it could reduce injuries? Why or why not?

COUNCIL ON EDUCATION FOR PUBLIC HEALTH FOUNDATIONAL KNOWLEDGE AND COMPETENCIES

Foundational Knowledge
Profession and Science of Public Health
- Explain the critical importance of evidence in advancing public health knowledge.

Foundational Competencies
Planning and Management to Promote Health
- Select methods to evaluate public health programs.

REFERENCES

1. Nelso SR. *Steel Drivin' Man: John Henry, the Untold Story of an American Legend.* 1st ed. New York: Oxford University Press; 2006.

2. Crum AJ, Langer EJ. Mind-set matters: exercise and the placebo effect. *Psychol Sci.* 2007;18(2):165–171. doi:10.1111/j.1467-9280.2007.01867.x

3. Swartz K, Musci RJ, Beaudry MB, et al. School-based curriculum to improve depression literacy among US Secondary school students: a randomized effectiveness trial. *Am J Public Health.* 2017;107:1970–1976. doi:10.2105/AJPH.2017.304088

4. Mutanski B, Parsons JT, Sullivan PS, et al. Biomedical and behavioral outcomes of keep it up! eHealth HIV Prevention Program RCT. *Am J Prev Med.* 2018;55(2):151–158. doi:10.1016/j.amepre.2018.04.026

5. Garrison KA, Pal P, O'Malley SS, et al. Craving to quit: a randomized controlled trial of smartphone app-based mindfulness training for smoking cessation. *Nicotine Tob Res.* 2018;22(3):324–331. doi:10.1093/ntr/nty126

6. Crosby R, Charnigo RJ, Salazar LF, et al. Enhancing condom use among black male youths: a randomized controlled trail. *Am J Public Health.* 2014;104:2219–2225. doi:10.2105/AJPH.2014.302131

7. Connor TS, Brookie KL, Carr AC, et al. Let them eat fruit! The effect of fruit and vegetable consumption on psychological well-being in young adults: a randomized controlled trial. *PLoS One.* 2017;12(2):e0171206. doi:10.1371/journal.pone.0171206

8. Chang A, Patberg E, Cueto V, et al. Community health workers, access to care, and service utilization among Florida Latinos: a randomized controlled trial. *Am J Public Health.* 2018;108:1249–1251. doi:10.2105/AJPH.2018.304542

9. United States Food and Drug Administration. Guidance for industry E 10 choice of control group and related issues in clinical trials. 2001. Accessed August 16, 2019. http://www.fda.gov/cder/guidance/index.htm

10. McMurray JJV, Packer M, Desai AS, et al. Angiotensin–neprilysin inhibition versus enalapril in heart failure. *N Engl J Med.* 2014;371(11):993–1004. doi:10.1056/NEJMoa1409077

11. Cram P, Fendrick AM, Inadomi J, et al. The impact of a celebrity promotional campaign on the use of colon cancer screening: the Katie Couric Effect. *JAMA Inter Med*. 2003;163(13):1601–1605. doi:10.1001/archinte.163.13.1601

12. McCambridge J, Wilton J, Elbourne DR. Systematic review of the Hawthorne effect: new concepts are needed to study research participation effects. *J Clin Epidemiol*. 2014;67(3):267–277. doi:10.1016/j.jclinepi.2013.08.015

ADDITIONAL READINGS AND RESOURCES

Banack HR, Kauffman JS. Does selection bias explain the obesity paradox among individuals with cardiovascular disease? *Ann Epidemiol*. 2015;25(5):342–349. doi:10.1016/j.annepidem.2015.02.008

Bell M, Kenward MG, Fairclough DL, Horton NJ. Differential dropout and bias in randomised controlled trials: when it matters and when it may not. *BMJ*. 2013;346:e8668. doi:10.1136/bmj.e8668

Naci H, Soumerai SB. History bias, study design, and the unfulfilled promise of pay-for-performance policies in health care. *Prev Chronic Dis*. 2016;13:160133. doi:10.5888/pcd13.160133externalicon

Trochim WMK. Web enter for social research methods: hybrid experimental designs. 2006. Accessed August 16, 2019. https://socialresearchmethods.net/kb/exphybrd.php

Quantitative Study Designs: Nonexperimental

Should parachutes be evaluated with randomized controlled trials?

—Gordon C. S. Smith and Jill P. Pell,
public health researchers

LEARNING OBJECTIVES

After reading this chapter, the reader will be able to

- Explain the difference between experimental and nonexperimental study designs.
- Define *quasi-experimental study*.
- Name and describe two types of quasi-experimental study design.
- Describe qualities of a cross-sectional study.
- Identify other nonexperimental study designs relevant to public health research.
- Explain the concept of external validity.

INTRODUCTION

Although experimental study designs are often considered the gold standard for rigorous research, for various reasons random assignment may not be possible in some public health research studies. In a 2003 *British Medical Journal* satirical paper by Smith and Pell, the authors conclude, "As with many health interventions intended to prevent ill health, the effectiveness of parachutes has not been subjected to rigorous evaluation by randomized controlled trials."[1] Who would agree to be in a study in which the researchers randomly assigned participants to wearing or not wearing a parachute when jumping out of an airplane? All joking aside, there may be ethical limitations to randomization. For example, in a study of safe infant sleep practices for the prevention of sudden infant death syndrome, a researcher could not ethically assign some babies to sleep in ways that might be unsafe just to adhere to the requirements of a randomized controlled trial (RCT).

Community-wide studies are common in public health research. According to the socioecological model, community environment and policies within those communities are important influences on health.[2] However, communities cannot be randomly selected to implement and adhere to, for example, clean-indoor air policies or sugar-sweetened beverage taxes. The policies may already exist, but the enactment or lack of policy within a community happens outside the realm of research. Researchers could not simply "tell" one community to implement a tobacco tax, and subsequently prevent a neighboring control community not to enact the same tax. The communities can still be studied in a way to contribute to the body of evidence related to the health impact of these policies, but the studies may be limited by the lack of true random-control assignment.

In addition to ethical and practicality issues, probability results from an RCT do not provide enough information to evaluate large-scale public health interventions.[3] Causality is just one part of overall evidence. Feasibility, applicability, and practice-based evidence are also important. Just because an RCT is not appropriate does not mean that topic of study is not worth the effort. There are several study designs, when rigorously conducted, that provide valuable evidence of effectiveness of public health programs, policies, and interventions.

QUASI-EXPERIMENTAL STUDY DESIGNS

Quasi-experimental studies are common in public health research. The main difference between experimental and quasi-experimental studies is the lack of random assignment of participants. Without this random assignment, the third criteria of causal inference may not be met, whereas the researcher cannot be certain the outcome (dependent variable) was not caused by some factor other than the independent variable. If quasi-experimental studies are conducted in ways that attempt to control for threats to interval validity, the results provide valuable information contributing to the body of evidence on the topic studied. There are two main quasi-experimental study designs commonly used in public health research studies. The **nonequivalent comparison groups design** is just like the experimental pretest–posttest control group design except without random participant assignment. It can be drawn as follows:

$$O_1 \quad X \quad O_2$$
$$O_1 \qquad\quad O_2$$

In this design, there are two groups. Both groups are assessed at baseline; one group is exposed to the intervention and the other is not. Both groups are measured again at posttest and the results are compared. Suppose, for example, you wanted to study the effect of providing extra recess to elementary students during the school day to increase physical activity. It is unlikely you would be able to randomly assign some students in a class to get an extra recess break without providing it to others in the same class. Perhaps you might be able to compare different classes within the same school, or compare classes located in different schools. In this type of study design, it is very important to assess comparability of groups at baseline. If the average physical activity level among students is about the same for both classes being compared, it would be reasonable to assume any differences at posttest would be due to the effect of the independent variable (extra recess). Other factors related to group comparison need to be taken into consideration as well. Sociodemographic factors, school characteristics, even gender of the class may alter comparability, thus limiting how certain we are of the effect of the independent variable. The researcher must document measures of comparability of the groups on any variable that theoretically or practically might influence the outcome.

PAID FAMILY LEAVE ON BREASTFEEDING: A QUASI-EXPERIMENTAL STUDY OF U.S. POLICIES

Research shows early return to work after childbirth is associated with reduced breastfeeding practices. A study by Hamad et al. provides a good example of quasi-experimental study design to evaluate the impact of policies on breastfeeding. The authors chose to evaluate breastfeeding outcomes from two states with enhanced paid family leave policies (California and New Jersey). Both states enacted policies allowing up to 6 weeks of partially paid leave. Researchers used breastfeeding data from the National Immunization Study and made comparisons of breastfeeding rates in the experimental group (California and New Jersey) with other states having no family leave policies. Rates were compared before (pretest) and after (posttest) the policies were enacted.[4] Random assignment was not possible due to the enactment of the states' breastfeeding policies. Nevertheless, findings from this quasi-experimental study are valuable to build the evidence for policy interventions to increase breastfeeding.

Another quasi-experimental study design is the **time series study design**. In this design, there are multiple pretests and multiple posttests. Time series is useful for understanding the process of how behaviors or factors change over time, or how interventions or policies influence these behaviors or factors. Time series can be depicted as:

$$O_1 \quad O_2 \quad O_3 \quad X \quad O_4 \quad O_5 \quad O_6$$

In this depiction, there are three measurements before the intervention and three after the intervention. This design is useful in studying the impact of policies. Suppose you are interested in exploring the impact of a new workplace clean-air policy. The new policy states that no one can smoke within 50 feet of a building entrance/exit. The management communicates the policy to employees 3 months before it goes into effect. Since you have time before the official policy starts, you can assess outdoor smoking behavior at three time points before the official implementation. You might observe the environment around the entrances during the first weeks of October, November, and December. If the policy takes place January 1, you can do another three assessments at 1-month intervals starting the first week of February. By analyzing the time series data, you may determine whether the policy is effective in moving smokers away from entrances/exits. By doing multiple measurements, you will be able to identify patterns in compliance. Maybe people who smoke will adhere to the policy at onset of implementation, but unless it is routinely enforced, they may slide back into smoking by the doors a few months after enactment. Time series is also useful to measure the sustainability of behavior change. If patterns emerge on reduction in behavioral improvement over time, longer interventions or more follow-ups may be recommended for future studies. It is up to the researcher to determine the appropriate number and time interval of assessments. Past literature and theory may help inform this planning.

Time series design with two groups is also commonly used in public health research. This design can be drawn as follows:

$$O_1 \quad O_2 \quad O_3 \quad X \quad O_4 \quad O_5 \quad O_6$$
$$O_1 \quad O_2 \quad O_3 \qquad O_4 \quad O_5 \quad O_6$$

Measures are conducted multiple times before and after an intervention in one group, and at the same time intervals for the control group without exposure to the intervention. This design is useful for studying behavior change resulting from interventions or policies. The use of two groups provides a check for some of the threats to internal validity of this quasi-experimental design, especially history. If an extraneous event occurs and impacts the outcome of interest, both groups would show change and the effect could not be attributed to the intervention being studied.

CROSS-SECTIONAL STUDY DESIGNS

Cross-sectional studies are widely used in public health research, particularly in exploratory or descriptive research. In these studies, the researcher examines a phenomenon by collecting and analyzing data from one point in time, or gets a "cross-sectional" view of the phenomenon. Surveys assessing a topic of interest at one point in time are cross-sectional. Suppose you are interested in gaining insight into the perception of community residents on the development of several new vaping retail stores. You can develop a survey that covers the breadth of the concept and send it out to all adults in the community of interest. This is an example of a cross-sectional study. Your results show age is negatively correlated with support for the vaping stores, whereas the older a person is the less likely they are to perceive the stores as good for the community. This correlation can provide valuable information on the topic of interest, but due to the nature of the cross-sectional study design, should be interpreted with caution. Unlike quasi-experimental study designs that attempt to reduce threats to internal validity, cross-sectional studies have internal validity limitations (see Figure 7.1). Remember, correlation is not causation. Causal inferences cannot be made from cross-sectional studies. Researchers can, however, attempt to rule out validity issues by using multivariate analytical techniques. You can strengthen your cross-sectional study by using a representative sample, sufficient sample size, and employing valid and reliable measures. These methods and controlling for alternative variables in analysis improves the study, but ultimately, the limits of cross-sectional studies remain.

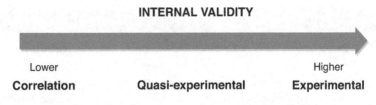

FIGURE 7.1 **Types of study design and internal validity.**

LONGITUDINAL STUDY DESIGNS

In **longitudinal studies**, there is a time order for data collection. By collecting data at different time points, researchers are able to determine whether the change in the independent variable precedes the change in the dependent variable. In public health research, these types of studies are useful when looking at changes in prevalence of behaviors or diseases over time. There are several different types of longitudinal studies. **Trend studies**, or repeated cross-sectional studies, are designed to capture data at two or more time points from different samples of the same population. The U.S. Census Current Population Survey[5] (CPS) is an example of a trend study. CPS data are the primary source of labor force statistics for the population of the United States. Data for topics such as poverty, health insurance coverage, and income are important factors for public health research. Because people come and go from populations of interest, it may be difficult to follow the exact group of people over the course of time. The U.S. Census Bureau collects CPS data from a sample of 60,000 households each month. Trend studies are appropriate for seeking information on the change of some phenomenon within populations over time. **Cohort studies** are longitudinal studies for which data are collected at two or more time points from individuals or groups with a common starting point (e.g., ninth grade in 2010). Birth cohorts, age cohorts, alumni cohorts, and employee cohorts are common population groups used in this type of longitudinal study. The Framingham Heart Study is a cohort study that began in 1948 to identify common factors or characteristics contributing to cardiovascular disease. The original cohort included 5,209 men and women between the ages of 30 and 62 from the town of Framingham, Massachusetts. Over the course of 70 years, five more cohorts have been added and data are collected from these groups on a regular basis.[6] **Panel studies** are longitudinal studies in which data are collected at two or more points in time from the same individuals, but unlike cohort studies, may not have a common starting point. Whereas trend studies explore population changes over time, panel studies focus on individual changes. The Medical Expenditure Panel Survey (MEPS) conducted by the U.S. Department of Health and Human Services Agency for Healthcare Research and Quality is a set of large-scale surveys of families and individuals, their medical providers, and employers across the United States.[7] Data are collected annually and inform healthcare and health insurance research and decision-making. Additional examples of longitudinal public health studies are shown in Table 7.1.

Although longitudinal studies provide valuable information on many public health topics, there are some challenges to implementing this type of study design. It is costly and time-consuming to keep track of people in cohort or panel studies. People move in and out of geographic areas, change phone numbers and emails, and may not update project staff with new information. Attrition among participants can also be a disadvantage. Analytical methods of longitudinal data should include comparison of characteristics of those who drop

TABLE 7.1 EXAMPLES OF LONGITUDINAL STUDIES IN PUBLIC HEALTH		
Study	**Description**	**Reference**
Nurses Health Study[10]	The Nurses Health Studies are among the largest prospective investigations into the risk factors for major chronic diseases in women. Starting with the original Nurses Health Study in 1976, the studies are now in their third generation with Nurses Health Study 3 (which is still enrolling male and female nurses) and count more than 275,000 participants.	www.nurseshealthstudy.org/about-nhs
Longitudinal Study of Aging (LSOA)[11]	The LSOAs is a collaborative project of NCHS and the NIA. It is a multicohort study of persons 70 years of age and over designed primarily to measure changes in the health, functional status, living arrangements, and health services utilization of two cohorts of Americans as they move into and through the oldest ages.	www.cdc.gov/nchs/lsoa/index.htm
National Longitudinal Study of Adolescent to Adult Health[12]	The National Longitudinal Study of Adolescent to Adult Health (Add Health), 1994–2008 [Public Use] is a longitudinal study of a nationally representative sample of U.S. adolescents in grades 7 through 12 during the 1994–1995 school year. The Add Health cohort was followed into young adulthood with four in-home interviews, the most recent conducted in 2008 when the sample was aged 24–32. Add Health combines longitudinal survey data on respondents' social, economic, psychological, and physical well-being with contextual data on the family, neighborhood, community, school, friendships, peer groups, and romantic relationships.	www.icpsr.umich.edu/icpsrweb/DSDR/studies/21600
The Infant Feeding Practices Study II[13]	IFPS II, conducted by the FDA and the CDC in 2005–2007, is a longitudinal study that followed about 2,000 mother–infant pairs from the third trimester of pregnancy throughout the first year of life to study a variety of infant feeding practices.	www.cdc.gov/breastfeeding/data/ifps/

(continued)

TABLE 7.1 EXAMPLES OF LONGITUDINAL STUDIES IN PUBLIC HEALTH (continued)		
Study	**Description**	**Reference**
Framingham Heart Study[6]	Since 1948, the Framingham Heart Study, under the direction of the NHLBI, formerly known as the *National Heart Institute*, has been committed to identifying the common factors or characteristics that contribute to CVD. It has followed CVD development over a long period of time in three generations of participants.	www.framinghamheartstudy.org/fhs-about/
National Longitudinal Survey of Public Health Systems[14]	Since 1998, researchers have followed a nationally representative cohort of U.S. communities to examine the types of public health activities performed within the community, the range of organizations contributing to each activity, and the perceived effectiveness of each activity in addressing community needs. This information, obtained through a validated survey of local public health officials, provides an in-depth view of the structure and function of local public health delivery systems and how these systems evolve over time.	www.publichealthsystems.org/national-longitudinal-survey-public-health-systems

CDC, Centers for Disease Control and Prevention; CVD, cardiovascular disease; FDA, Food and Drug Administration; IFPS II, Infant Feeding Practices Study II; LSOAs, Longitudinal Studies of Aging; NCHS, National Center for Health Statistics; NHLBI, National Heart, Lung and Blood Institute; NIA, National Institute on Aging.

out of a study and those who remain to justify the integrity of the final data. Also,participants in longitudinal studies with many data-collection points may experience subject fatigue in which they grow weary of repeatedly being asked for information or participation. Proper incentives and easing participant burden are vital for successful longitudinal studies.

OTHER NONEXPERIMENTAL QUANTITATIVE STUDY DESIGNS

Research opportunities can be unpredictable. Sometimes you may not be able to prepare for or implement the best and most rigorous study design. There are other study designs with low internal validity, which can be used for topic exploration or to inform other more rigorous studies. These are sometimes called *preexperimental designs*. The **one-shot case study** is a design in which measurement of one group takes place after an intervention. There is no covariation, baseline measurement, or comparison group. This design is drawn as:

X   O

Without a pretest measure or a comparison group, there is a possibility of the outcome being attributable to some other extraneous variable and not just the intervention, so you cannot infer causality. This study design might be useful to explore perceptions, behaviors, or practices after a natural disaster or some sort of unexpected occurrence for which no baseline data was be collected prior to the event. For example, a researcher might be interested in studying how a highly publicized food-borne illness outbreak from tainted lettuce might impact purchasing of vegetables by community residents. Surveys can assess self-reported change in purchasing behavior and perceptions of food safety. Although there is no certainty any change in purchasing behavior is solely due to the outbreak, the information from the study can be added to other data on the topic or inform future studies. Publication of data from one-shot case studies must include the important limitations to data interpretation.

Another study design without the rigor of experimental or quasi-experimental strategies is the **one-group pretest–posttest**. This design can be depicted:

$$O_1 \quad x \quad O_2$$

Unlike the one-shot case study, there is a baseline measurement before and after the intervention. Because there can be comparisons of these two measurements, the research can explore covariation. However, the design has low internal validity, mainly due to the threats of history, maturation, and testing. Without a comparison group, there is no certainty the outcome may not be due to some other factor. Sometimes this type of study is done out of convenience. For example, master's of public health (MPH) students can be surveyed about their preventive health behaviors at the beginning of the program and the end of the program. This data will provide information on behavioral change within the MPH student population, but you cannot be sure the knowledge gained throughout the program of study influenced this change.

The **posttest-only with nonequivalent groups** design is drawn:

$$X \quad O$$
$$O$$

This design takes the one-shot case study design and adds a comparison group, both only measured at posttest. Because there is no random assignment, there is no way of knowing whether the groups are comparable. In the food-borne illness and vegetable-purchasing example previously discussed, a researcher using the posttest-only with nonequivalent groups may choose to survey residents in a community not exposed to or affected by the outbreak in addition to the group in the community where the outbreak occurred. Although it may be considered better than a one-shot case study, this design has low internal validity due to the potential for selection bias. The researcher has no way of knowing how much the groups differed in purchasing behavior prior to the outbreak event.

Single-case study designs are less common in public health than other fields such as psychology or social work. In these study designs, an individual is assessed on the dependent variable multiple times prior to and after the intervention. The multiple data points show trends and sustainability of intervention outcomes. Figure 7.2 depicts one way data from a single-case study can be graphed. In this example, a single participant (a teenage mother of a toddler) is in a counseling program. She is assessed on several psychological factors each week, including perceived stress. Her counselor feels as if an intervention is needed to reduce stress. (A) shows baseline (or control) measures of her stress each week for 5 weeks and (B)

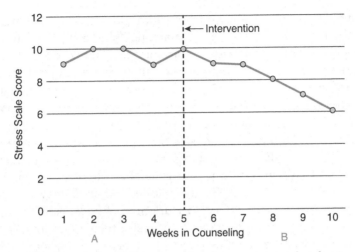

FIGURE 7.2 **Example of data from a single-case study design.**

shows the trend in stress scores following the intervention (weeks 6–10). You can see the trend in the reduction of stress score for weeks after the intervention. The multiple measures reduce the threats to internal validity, but factors, such as history, may still be a limitation. Some studies of this type use more than one baseline and intervention phase. If the trend is in the desired direction during the intervention phases, but not the baseline phases, there is more evidence to demonstrate history may not be a threat to the study's internal validity.

EXTERNAL VALIDITY

Public health research findings would be of little use if the results have limited application to broader populations or settings. When a study has high internal validity, there is assurance of the causal inferences of the study findings between the setting and sample. **External validity** is the extent to which a study's findings are applicable or generalizable to other populations and settings. There are two main types of external validity: population and ecological. **Population external validity** refers to how well the research on a sample can be generalized to other samples or the whole population. If your study sample were a group of adolescents, would the results be generalizable to all adolescents? Population external validity can be tricky. If your study sample is Hispanic women of childbearing age, your results may not be generalizable to Hispanic women in other age groups or women of other races/ethnicities. You may even have trouble justifying your findings as representative of all Hispanic women of childbearing age, especially in the context of setting. The second type of external validity is **ecological external validity**. This type pertains to how well the results can be generalized to other settings or contexts. For example, if your study results identify specific correlates of physical activity for adults in an urban community, would those correlates be generalizable to suburban or rural settings? The level to which your study findings can be generalized to other populations, settings, or contexts should align with your overall study goals.

Perfect external validity in a study is unlikely as there are several factors that challenge it.[8] The threats to external validity are somewhat similar to those affecting internal validity. One threat is the testing effect. In studies with pretests or baseline measures, the mere act of the testing may affect performance of participants in a research study. Results may not be generalizable to situations without pretesting. Using a Solomon four-group design can reduce the risk of this threat because you can compare those with and without pretesting. Another threat to external validity is the potential interaction among "treatments" or intervention components. This interaction may contribute to the outcome. For example, maybe it is not the dietary changes or the physical activity that improves overall cardiovascular risk, but a combination of the two. A third challenge to generalizability is selection bias. The characteristics of the participants selected for the study may interact with the treatment or intervention components, subsequently influencing the outcome. As stated previously, a large, random sample will reduce the chances for this bias and thus improve external validity. Fourth, simply knowing a research study is being implemented (e.g., Hawthorne effect) may impact the outcome and reduce the extent to which results may be generalized to other populations or settings. Last, the ways in which concepts are defined and tested in a study may reduce the likelihood of generalizability. For example, the term "leisure-time physical activity" did not resonate with women in one study because they did not perceive themselves to have "leisure time."[9] Looking to past literature and conducting pilot tests of measures may help reduce this threat.

It is important to design public health research studies in ways that achieve the best possible external validity. In addition, because evidence is an aggregate of research findings, factors related to external validity need to be reported in the literature. This will to help others conducting related studies and improve translation of findings into public health practice. Steckler and McLeroy[8] suggest the following items are necessary to include when reporting study results:

- recruitment procedures,
- participation and attrition rates,
- sample representativeness,
- settings,
- implementation consistency,
- importance of outcomes to a variety of audiences, and
- sustainability and long-term effects.

Although not all of these components are relevant to every public health research study, more thorough reporting will improve the ability to generalize research results more broadly. Better reporting will also improve the ways in which policy and decision-makers understand the applicability of research findings within their context. When research is translated into practice, population health benefits.

CHAPTER DISCUSSION QUESTIONS

1. How would you justify your quasi-experimental study design to a group of medical researchers who think RCT studies are the only way to do research?
2. What are the pros and cons of time series with a control group and a nonequivalent control group design to study the impact of a new healthy-eating portion of a health education curriculum taught to third-grade students?
3. Why is the cross-sectional study design so common in public health research?
4. How could you enhance the external validity of your nonequivalent control group study to compare the impact of a media campaign on the negative health impacts of initiating vaping for adolescents?

RESEARCH PROJECT CHECK-IN

Thinking About Study Design

There is a good chance you will use a nonexperimental study design for your course research project, based on access to study populations and timing of a semester-long course. What is the most appropriate nonexperimental design for your topic? List out some benefits and limitations of at least two different designs, and choose the one that fits best with your research topic. Also, begin to think about external validity. How might you enhance the generalizability of your findings?

PUBLIC HEALTH RESEARCH METHODS IN REAL LIFE

Random Alternatives

Many stakeholders are interested in the benefits of creating walkable neighborhoods. There is some evidence on reduced injuries, more social capital, and increased physical activity of residents who live in places with sidewalks. Before investing in a neighborhood sidewalk improvement program, the mayor of a suburban town wants data on these benefits. She looks to the local pedestrian advocacy group to help design a study to get this data. Gina works for the advocacy agency, has her MPH degree, and is well trained to design and implement the study. In their first meeting to talk about the study, the mayor mentioned that she knows a little bit about research and asked Gina if an RCT would work.

Street and sidewalk improvements were happening around town as part of usual transportation maintenance. The order in which they were done was established by the transportation department and related to the age of the existing infrastructure as well as the extent of the improvements needed. It would not be possible to randomize people to live in neighborhoods with sidewalks and without, but the study could still be done in a rigorous way. Gina decided to propose two different ways to study this issue. The first was a quasi-experimental study in which baseline walking behavior would be assessed for all residents in a neighborhood before improvements were made and after the sidewalks were improved. Because the projects were happening on a rolling basis, members of the control group would all be residents in neighborhoods that were planned for improvement the following year. This design would still provide useful data comparing the neighborhood influence on walking behavior.

The second study design Gina proposed was a time series design without a control group. In this design she would assess a sample of residents in all the neighborhoods with upcoming sidewalk improvement projects prior to project commencement, then 1 month, 3 months, and 6 months after the projects were completed. Differences and sustainability of walking behavior changes could be shown with the data.

Gina presented both options to the mayor and explained that either would provide data on walking behavior before and after sidewalk improvements. The time series would also shed light on the longer term impact on walking. Both designs had pros and cons. Neither design would determine causality because of lack of random assignment and the chance that some factor other than the sidewalk improvement would influence the outcome. The mayor was not satisfied with the proposed designs and asked Gina to develop one more. She suggested a hybrid design, using the best of both of the studies Gina proposed.

Gina thought about issues, such as timing, resources, and feasibility, when figuring out this new study design. She also learned that she needed to provide data to the advocacy agency within 2 years in order for funds for the enhanced sidewalk improvement program to be included in the next-cycle budget. The new study design was a quasi-experimental time series design with a control group. She selected three neighborhoods that were on the transportation department calendar for sidewalk improvements in the next 6 months. Each project was slated to take 3 months. She found three control neighborhoods in line for improvements to community sidewalks, but not until 2 fiscal years from the current point in time. She would assess residents on walking behavior at baseline, then at 1, 3, and 6 months after project completion. This would give her time to collect data in the control groups before their neighborhood sidewalk improvements started. The mayor appreciated this design and gave approval to further develop the study.

Critical Thinking Questions

1. How could a neighborhood study like this be crafted into an experimental design study?
2. What are some threats to internal validity that might be present in both of the proposed designs? Was her final hybrid design less likely to have these threats? Why or why not?
3. What are some of the benefits of doing a time series design for a study like this? Multiple measurements take more time and resources. Do the benefits outweigh these disadvantages?
4. How would you inform someone (like the mayor in this story) that random design is not always the best approach?
5. What are the pros and cons of measuring everyone in a neighborhood versus only a sample of residents?

COUNCIL ON EDUCATION FOR PUBLIC HEALTH FOUNDATIONAL KNOWLEDGE AND COMPETENCES

Foundational Knowledge
Profession and Science of Public Health
- Explain the critical importance of evidence in advancing public health knowledge.

Foundational Competencies
Planning and Management to Promote Health
- Select methods to evaluate public health programs.

REFERENCES

1. Smith GCS, Pell JP. Parachute use to prevent death and major trauma related to gravitational challenge: systematic review of randomised controlled trials. *BMJ.* 2003;327(7429):1459–1461. doi:10.1136/bmj.327.7429.1459

2. McLeroy KR, Bibeau D, Steckler A, et al. An ecological perspective on health promotion programs. *Health Educ Q.* 1988;15(4):351–377. Accessed September 9, 2019. https://www.academia.edu/170661/An_Ecological_Perspective_on_Health_Promotion_Programs

3. Victora CG, Habicht JP, Bryce J. Evidence-based public health: moving beyond randomized trials. *Am J Public Health.* 2004;94(3):400–405. doi:10.2105/ajph.94.3.400

4. Hamad R, Modrek S, White J. Paid family leave effects on breastfeeding: a quasi-experimental study of US policies. *Am J Public Health.* 2019;109(1):164–165. doi:10.2105/AJPH.2018.304693

5. U.S. Census Bureau. Current population survey (CPS). 2018. Accessed September 11, 2019. https://www.census.gov/programs-surveys/cps.html

6. Framingham Heart Study. About the Framingham heart study. 2019. Accessed September 11, 2019. https://www.framinghamheartstudy.org/fhs-about/

7. U.S. Department of Health and Human Services, Agency for Healthcare Research and Quality. Medical expenditure panel survey home. 2019. Accessed September 11, 2019. https://www.meps.ahrq.gov/mepsweb

8. Steckler A, McLeroy KR. The importance of external validity. *Am J Public Health.* 2008;98(1):9–10. doi:10.2105/AJPH.2007.126847

9. Eyler AA, Baker E, Cromer L, et al. Physical activity and minority women: a qualitative study. *Health Educ Behav.* 1998;25(5):640–652. doi:10.1177/109019819802500510

10. Bao Y, Bertoia ML, Lenart EB, et al. Origin, methods, and evolution of the Three Nurses' Health Studies. *Am J Public Health.* 2016;106(9):1573–1581. doi:10.2105/AJPH.2016.303338

11. National Center for Health Statistics. The Longitudinal Study of Aging. 2019. Accessed September 5, 2020. http://www.cdc.gov/nchs/lsoa/index.htm

12. Harris KM, Udry JR. National Longitudinal Study of Adolescent to Adult Health (Add Health), 1994–2008 [Public Use]. Carolina Population Center, University of North Carolina-Chapel Hill [distributor], Inter-university Consortium for Political and Social Research [distributor]. August 6, 2018. doi:10.3886/ICPSR21600.v21

13. Centers for Disease Control and Prevention. Infant Feeding Practices Study II. 2018. Accessed September 5, 2020. http://www.cdc.gov/breastfeeding/data/ifps/

14. Robert Wood Johnson Foundation. National Longitudinal Survey of Public Health Systems. 2020. Accessed September 5, 2020. http://www.publichealthsystems.org/national-longitudinal-survey-public-health-systems

ADDITIONAL READINGS AND RESOURCES

Bärnighausen T, Røttingen JA, Rockers P, et al. Quasi-experimental study designs series—paper 1: introduction: two historical lineages. *J Clin Epidemiol*. 2017;89:4–11. doi:10.1016/j.jclinepi.2017.02.020

Puddy RW, Wilkins N. *Understanding Evidence Part 1: Best Available Research Evidence. A Guide to the Continuum of Evidence of Effectiveness*. Atlanta, GA: Centers for Disease Control and Prevention; 2011.

Developing Budgets and Timelines for Research Studies

Plan what you can afford.
—National Institute of Allergy and Infectious Diseases,
grant budget guidance

LEARNING OBJECTIVES

After reading this chapter, the reader will be able to

- Describe how public health research is funded.
- Identify and define the components of a research budget.
- Write a budget justification.
- Name and describe two types of research granting agencies.
- Describe differences between federal and nonprofit research grants.
- Identify components to consider when planning timeline and budgets.
- Develop a realistic research project timeline.

INTRODUCTION

Over the past century, medical and public health research has made great contributions to improvements in population health and added decades to life expectancy.[1] Two key aspects of successful research are innovative ideas and financial support. Once you come up with your innovate research idea, the next step is to navigate potential funding sources and clearly articulate the approach and costs of your prosed project. Acquiring money for public health research is very competitive. In 2018, only 21% of applications received by the National Institutes of Health (NIH), the main source for public health research, were successful in being funded.[2] Why is it so difficult to get research money? First, the economics of public health research are grim. Government and other funding priorities change over time, and public health funding is often a target when budget cuts become necessary. Second, healthcare spending takes precedence over prevention. Medical care produces much more visible results than prevention research. It is sometimes difficult to sell an unseen concept such as the number of heart attacks prevented from evidence-based public health efforts.[3] In addition, the improvements in health might take a long time to occur so the investment in research may seem less of a priority than other more current issues.

No matter what the goals of your public health career may be, understanding funding and budgets is necessary knowledge. The national accrediting body of public health education, the Council on Education for Public Health (CEPH), included this topic as one of the Master of Public Health Foundational Competencies. Beginning in 2016, public health curricula are required to include educational components on the basic principles and tools of budget and resource management.[4]

FUNDERS OF PUBLIC HEALTH RESEARCH

International Funding Agencies

There are several different categories of funding sources for public health research. In the United States, government agencies are the largest financial sponsor of public health research. Globally, countries differ in the mechanisms of prioritizing, funding, and monitoring health research studies. Multicountry organizations, such as the European Commission or the Pan American Health Organization, provide opportunities for research funding.[5] There are also international alliances, which fund research related to specific topics such as the Global Alliance for Vaccines or the Global Fund to Fight AIDS.[5] The World Health Organization (WHO) is an agency within the United Nations, and is the largest multicountry alliance to promote health. The WHO manages funding from multiple governments and voluntary contributions. One aspect of the WHO's mission to promote worldwide health is to use research, evidence, and information as the foundation for health policies. The WHO supports research with the following goals[6]:

- Build capacity to strengthen health research systems.
- Support health priorities in middle and low-income countries.
- Create norms and standards of good research practice.
- Ensure quality evidence is translated into affordable health technologies and evidence-informed policy.

The WHO has many research groups, ranging in topical focus from influenza and vaccine research to health policy and health systems. More information on WHO research can be found at www.who.int/health-topics/research/.

Federal Research Funding

In the United States, the amount of government research funding is dependent on the annual federal budget. The process starts with budget requests from all federal departments. The president reviews and summarizes the requests and submits a full budget request to Congress. Federal agencies, such as the Congressional Budget Office, provide oversight and recommendations. Congress creates and approves a new federal budget each year, and the president ultimately signs the budget into law or vetoes it and the process continues. Appropriations bills designate the amounts allocated to agencies and programs. Within the agencies and programs, priorities for medical or public health research may not always be proportional to the disease burden.[7] The health issues that are the most prevalent may not always get the most funding. Also, just like people in elected offices, budgets and political priorities can change, affecting the research agenda.

Government-funded research plays an important role in developing evidence-based strategies to prevent diseases and improve health. Health services research is the broad category that encompasses examination of access to care; care cost and quality; and the health and well-being of individuals, communities, and populations. However, health services research receives only 0.3% of total healthcare expenditures or only 1/20th of science funding.[8] In 2010, the Affordable Care Act established the Prevention and Public Health Fund to provide investments in public health, including research.[9] Money from this fund goes to community and clinical prevention initiatives, research, surveillance, immunizations and screening, tobacco prevention, and public health workforce and infrastructure. In the Consolidated Appropriations Act of 2012, Congress required the Department of Health and Human Services (HHS) to establish a website for reporting on uses of funds made available through the Prevention and Public Health Fund.[9]

Although several U.S. governmental departments are involved in public health research (Table 8.1), the HHS oversees the agencies most likely to be sources of public health research funding. Much of public health research funding comes from NIH and the Centers for Disease Control and Prevention (CDC), but other divisions, such as Substance Abuse and Mental Health Services Administration (SAMHSA), and Agency for Healthcare Research and Quality (AHRQ), may also be sources of funding. This section focuses on the NIH and CDC as main federal funding agencies for public health research.

TABLE 8.1 EXAMPLES OF U.S. FEDERAL AGENCIES PARTNERING WITH HEALTH AND HUMAN SERVICES TO FUND PUBLIC HEALTH RESEARCH

U.S. Government Agency	Example of Public Health Research
United States Department of Agriculture (USDA)	USDA has a research action plan that identified seven priorities, including global food supply, nutrition and childhood obesity, and food safety. For more information about this example, see www.usda.gov/topics/research-and-science
Department of Defense (DOD)	The DOD and the individual branches of the military sponsor research related to physical and psychological health of military members and their families. Example: mrdc.amedd.army.mil/index.cfm/program_areas/medical_research_and_development

(continued)

TABLE 8.1 EXAMPLES OF U.S. FEDERAL AGENCIES PARTNERING WITH HEALTH AND HUMAN SERVICES TO FUND PUBLIC HEALTH RESEARCH *(continued)*

U.S. Government Agency	Example of Public Health Research
Department of Education (DOE)	DOE provides funding through the National Center for Education Research. Grant topics include promotion of student mental health and well-being, development of effective health curricula, and promoting healthy sleep habits. ies.ed.gov/funding/20rfas.asp
Housing and Urban Development (HUD)	HUD provides research funding for topics such as healthy and safe homes and neighborhood planning. www.hud.gov/program_offices/spm/gmomgmt/grantsinfo/fundingopps
Department of Transportation (DOT)	DOT provides funds for research on safe streets, active transportation, public transit, safe routes to school, and the recreational trail program. www.transportation.gov/bicycles-pedestrians
Department of Labor (DOL)	DOL leads the Occupational Safety and Health Administration, which provides funding for studies pertaining to preventing injuries and diseases, as well as promoting employee health. www.osha.gov/dte/sharwood
Veterans Affairs (VA)	The VA has several mechanisms for funding public health research, including health services research and development and the Center for Health Equity Research and Promotion. www.hsrd.research.va.gov/funding/apply.cfm

National Institutes of Health

The NIH is the main medical and public health research agency in the United States. It is made up of 27 different institutes and centers, each with a specific focus (e.g., disease or bodily system) and its own research agenda. For example, the National Institute of Diabetes and Digestive and Kidney Diseases (NIDDK) funds research on chronic diseases such as diabetes, but also prioritizes nutrition and obesity studies as part of disease prevention. A full list of institutes and research priorities is available (www.nih.gov/institutes-nih/list-nih-institutes-centers-offices). Within the NIH, the Office of the Director is responsible for prioritizing, planning, managing, and coordinating programs within the 27 institutes and centers. In 2019, the NIH funded $39 billion in research through almost 50,000 competitive grants at more than 2,500 universities, medical schools, or research institutions. In order to facilitate public accountability of use of federal money, the NIH has a system of reporting in which anyone can access information on all funded research activities along with the results of supported research (e.g., detailed reports of annual research funding by category or disease).[7]

NATIONAL INSTITUTES OF HEALTH GRANT RESEARCH PROCESS

By this time in your public health studies, you probably have heard of or even participated in grant research. Have you ever wondered how it all works? The process of grant research is arduous and sometimes excruciating, but can be very rewarding. When a health researcher has an idea for a research project, the researcher often looks to the NIH for funding opportunities. Sometimes there is a specific request for proposal (RFP), pProgram announcement (PA), or funding opportunity announcement (FOA) that outlines detailed topics and requirements for grant projects. These typically arise from one of the 27 institutes within the NIH, such as the National Cancer Institute (NCI) or National Heart, Lung, and Blood Institute (NHLBI). Funding opportunities can be found on the NIH website. There are different types of grants available from the NIH, with the RO1 research grant category being the largest and most well funded at $500,000 per year for 5 years. Academic research careers are often built on the ability to achieve RO1 funding. Other smaller grants, such as the R21 and RO3, are also commonly used for public health research. These are funded at a lower amount and are shorter in duration than the RO1, but not any easier to get. See grants. nih.gov/grants/funding/funding_program.htm for a full list of types of grant programs.

Once you choose to apply for one of the funding opportunities or submit a grant idea outside of one of the FOAs, the first step is to become very familiar with the instructions. NIH requires very specific information and not adhering to the guidelines will result in an unsuccessful application. There is likely a university research office that can help you with the grant logistics. Most NIH grants operate on a regular submission schedule with application deadlines in February, June, and October. When the grant is written and all necessary ancillary material is submitted, you wait ... and wait. If you submit your grant in October, you will be notified of review status the following March, and funding status by May.

Your application will be assigned to a study section. The study section is made up of qualified reviewers with the expertise needed to critically judge the merits of your proposal. Your application will be reviewed by three members of the study section, and given a score from 1 to 9 for different categories (e.g., innovation, approach), with 1 being the best score and 9 being the worst. Scores are averaged. Researchers with proposals in the bottom half of all applications reviewed by the study section receive written feedback from reviewers. The top half are presented in order during an in-person study section meeting, discussed, and scored. The score from this meeting is what determines the overall rank and prioritization for funding. Currently, proposals only in the top 10% to 15% get funding.

Centers for Disease Control and Prevention

The CDC is an operating component of the HHS. It implements programs and conducts research to build evidence, inform practice, and works to translate this research for improved population health. The CDC uses grants and cooperative agreements to fund research and nonresearch public health programs and practices. Centers within the CDC include Occupational Safety and Health, Public Health Science and Surveillance, Noninfectious Diseases, and Infectious Diseases. In 2019, the CDC spent almost $6.5 billion for programming and research.[10] One of the ways the CDC sponsors public health research is through the Prevention Research Centers (PRC) Program (see www.cdc.gov/prc). The 25 PRCs are housed in universities with schools of public health or preventive medicine residencies. Researchers at PRCs conduct studies to identify, develop, and implement effective public health prevention strategies to help prevent chronic diseases. Research topics within the PRCs include aging, cancer, HIV and sexual health, obesity, physical activity, nutrition, epilepsy, and tobacco use.

State and Local Government Research Funding

State agencies can be a source of funding for public health research. Federal funds are often allocated to states, and the state agencies are responsible for distributing the money. For example, federal transportation funds are proportionally provided to each state. Part of these funds can go to programs and infrastructure that support walking and bicycling. Some state agencies have a competitive grant process they use to distribute funds. Community or regional agencies could apply for project-specific funding from the state. Just as with federal grant applications, these agencies must demonstrate the plan and capacity to spend funds appropriately, and are often judged against one another using some kind of predetermined prioritization. State health departments also are the recipients of federal money for programming and research. Researchers can partner with the state agencies and other stakeholders to create rigorous studies to help build the evidence for best practices. Local health departments, regional offices, and municipal governments can all be potential funding sources for

WHAT IS A RESEARCH UNIVERSITY?

Colleges and universities are one category of recipients of research funding. Doctoral students use research funding for attainment of their degree and career enhancement. The Carnegie Classification of Institutions of Higher Education is a list of the similarities and differences among institutions, and is used to rank research activity. From those schools recognized as doctoral-degree granting institutions, 131 were categorized in 2019 as R1 Doctoral Universities—indicating the highest research activity—and 135 institutions that are classified as R2 Doctoral Universities, indicating high research activity. The ranking also considers staff and expenditures related to research and development in this ranking. To put it simply, the R1 institutions demonstrate the best capacity for research activity. This ranking is often a consideration when choosing a place for doctoral studies.

Source: Center for Post-Secondary Research. The Carnegie Classification of Institutions of Higher Education. 2018. Accessed September 5, 2020. http://carnegieclassifications.iu.edu.

public health research. These opportunities are often highly collaborative, with many agencies and partners involved. Funding for collaborative projects of this type is typically smaller than federal grants and may come from multiple sources (e.g., a combination of state, local, and community agency funds). Being involved with state and local public health efforts is a way to be informed of these research opportunities.

Nonprofit Organizations as Funders of Public Health Research

"Nonprofit" is a legal organizational designation for which certain conditions must be met (e.g., not paying out profits to private shareholders or individuals) to be exempt from paying federal income taxes.[11] Private foundations and public charities are examples of nonprofit organizations. A nonprofit designated by the U.S. tax code as 501c3, can accept tax-deductible donations to use as part of their budget. These organizations can be national such as the American Heart Association or American Cancer Society, state based, or locally focused. Sometimes they are dedicated to specific topics (e.g., Susan G. Komen Breast Cancer Foundation). Others are broader in scope (e.g., the Kresge Foundation). Nonprofit organizations depend on research to help advance their public policy and public awareness initiatives.

Foundations are one category of nonprofit organizations that fund public health research. **Foundations** are nonprofit organizations donating funds to support other organizations or provide the source of funding for its own charitable purposes. In 2015, there were over 86,000 foundations registered in the United States.[12] Many corporations have affiliate (but legally designated as separate) foundations. Corporate foundations get funds from the profit-making company, usually sourced through investment income, donations, or endowment. The scope of the research funded by foundations is aligned specifically with its mission, and sometimes can be limited to geographic service areas of the parent corporation. Foundations typically provide smaller amounts of grant funding than the federal government, but can be a good source for pilot projects or smaller research studies. There are publicly available foundation directories that outline the specificity of research they fund. Universities may have staff to assist with foundation-funded research opportunities. Table 8.2 lists examples of foundations and the public health research they fund.

TABLE 8.2 EXAMPLES OF FOUNDATIONS AND PUBLIC HEALTH RESEARCH FUNDING	
Foundation	**Public Health Research Funding**
Aetna Foundation www.aetna-foundation.org	Opportunities include Cultivating Healthy Communities program to support healthy lifestyles in places where we live, work, learn, play, and pray.
Baxter International www.baxter.com/our-story/ fueling-collaborative-innovation/ research-continuing-education-grants	Baxter focuses funding on access to healthcare, community improvement, and scientific innovation.

(continued)

TABLE 8.2 EXAMPLES OF FOUNDATIONS AND PUBLIC HEALTH RESEARCH FUNDING (*continued*)	
Foundation	**Public Health Research Funding**
RWJF www.rwjf.org	RWJF funds a wide array of research and initiatives for new and innovative approaches to building a culture of health.
William T. Grant Foundation wtgrantfoundation.org/grants	This organization's mission is to improve everyday settings for youths, such as families, peer groups, schools, and neighborhoods.
WK Kellogg Foundation www.wkkf.org	This foundation is focused on overall health and well-being of children, especially related to health disparities.
State health foundations such as Missouri Foundation for Health mffh.org Colorado Health Foundation www.coloradohealth.org Georgia Health Foundation gahealthfdn.org Rhode Island Foundation rifoundation.org New York State Health Foundation nyshealthfoundation.org	State health foundations vary in scope and priority, but can be a good source for public health research funds, especially when projects are collaborations with state or community partners.

RWJF, Robert Wood Johnson Foundation.

Business and Industry

Many sectors of business and industry contribute to health research funding. The funding often comes from the affiliate foundation, with the focus area tied to the corporation's business interests. For example, a pharmaceutical company may provide public health research funding opportunities related to disease management and the drugs they produce (e.g., diabetes management). The scientific or clinical requirements for pharmaceutical funding are often accompanied by translational or equity components, which fit well with the skill set of a public health researcher. Funding can also come from other business sectors such as healthcare, agriculture, and technology. Funding and partnerships with industry can be advantageous, but may result in an unethical conflict of interest (Exhibit 8.1).

DEVELOPING A RESEARCH BUDGET

A research budget quantitatively outlines the required costs and financial plan for project-related expenses. A detailed and accurate budget helps identify and justify the financial

EXHIBIT 8.1 COCA-COLA FUNDING FOR OBESITY RESEARCH

Research funding from business and industry is not uncommon, but public health researchers should know that sometimes companies can use scientific research to their advantage, creating an ethical conflict. If a business funds a study, the research contract may often include provisions allowing the company to review and control the results of the funded studies. Imagine what a detriment it would be for a company, banking on profits from sugar-sweetened beverages, to get exposed for contributing to childhood obesity and all its consequences!

In 2015, the Coca-Cola Company gave $1 million to the University of Colorado Foundation to fund a research institute to study energy balance and obesity prevention—but really to shift the focus from calories consumed to exercise. The researcher leading the institute (James O. Hill) is a diet and nutrition expert who is well experienced with food-industry funding. However, when Coca-Cola's influence on the scientific research discussion on prevention of obesity was exposed, the university returned the $1 million gift due to ethical conflict.[16,17]

The issue is bigger than the returned funds. Industry-funded research could affect policy making by influencing the type of evidence available and the kinds of public health solutions considered. In a 2019 article published in the *Millbank Quarterly*, Maani Hessari and colleagues gained access to communications between Coca-Cola and the CDC. The review of these communications revealed efforts by Coca-Cola to "advance corporate objectives, rather than health."[13] This publication and ensuing negative exposure resulted in Coca-Cola modifying how it provides support for scientific research on well-being.

Are public health researchers missing out on innovative research projects by shunning industry funding? There are still ways to conduct ethical studies in collaboration with industry. Top research institutes require researchers to follow strict conflict-of-interest guidelines, and most have committees dedicated to reviewing and supervising conflicted research.

support needed for project implementation. Research budgets are complex, and there are several steps involved in developing one. The first essential step is to read through the rules and requirements of the funding agency. Many organizations, including the federal government, have very specific policies on the way in which research funds can and cannot be used. Most proposal guidance documents will outline these rules. One organizational factor paramount to preparing the budget is the designation of direct and indirect costs. **Direct costs** are costs directly related to the project, which can be assigned to project activities with a high degree of accuracy. Salary of the principal investigator (PI) and the research team is a direct cost. **Indirect costs** are sometimes called overhead or facilities and administration costs. These costs are not specifically aligned (i.e., indirectly related) to a specific project or activity, but are necessary for the general operation of the organization receiving the grant funds. Examples of indirect costs are space-related costs such as utilities, network costs, and salaries of support personnel. Universities assess the shared costs of research activity, and determine a percentage applied to each grant. For federal health grants, universities negotiate this percentage with the HHS. This set percentage needs to be factored into the total research budget as indirect costs. For example, if direct project costs are $300,000 and the indirect rate is 50%, $150,000 is calculated as the total for indirect costs incurred as a result of the project. The total amount awarded from the agency will be $450,000. For multiyear projects, the anticipated increase in the indirect rate needs to be considered in the budget. Check with your university research office to find out the indirect rate. Some funding organizations or foundations limit the percentage of indirect costs. The Robert Wood Johnson Foundation specifies its 2019 indirect rate as 12% of all costs associated with the project.[14] For research within U.S. universities and colleges, the maximum indirect costs rate for projects funded by the Bill and Melinda Gates Foundation is 10%.[15] Federal research grants provide more money to the institutions than the lower indirect rates offered with foundation funding.

After reading all the funding rules and budget requirements, make a list of all project activities, along with realistic costs related to conducting those activities. Suppose one of the project activities is implementing a survey by mail. What items would need to be included in the budget? Printing, postage, reminder cards, and envelopes would all be budget items. If participants are to return the completed survey via mail, return postage is also needed. Are you providing incentives for survey respondents? The amount and estimated number needed should be factored into the budget. In this example, look to past literature or pilot studies to estimate the response rate. You will only need to budget for the percentage likely to respond.

Budget guidance documents typically outline the ways the budget should be organized. Most proposals require broad categories such as personnel, materials and supplies, and travel. The personnel section outlines key people conducting project activities. The head of the project is called the PI. There can be other investigators, project managers, and research staff included in this section. The PI estimates the percentage of time each person will spend on the project. Suppose a PI will spend 15% of their work time (sometimes called full-time equivalent or FTE) on the proposed research project. Fifteen percent of this person's salary, plus the cost of fringe benefits, will be included in the personnel budget. For multiyear projects, increases in salary or hourly pay need to be considered. Federal grants have a salary cap, or limit on the amount of direct salary an individual may earn (see grants.nih.gov/grants/guide/notice-files/NOT-OD-19-099.html). The personnel costs often take up the majority of a grant budget. Consultant services do not fall under personnel costs, but are a separate budget category.

The materials and supplies section of the budget include consumable items needed for the project. For instance, this section would include the cost of specialized envelopes for mailing surveys or digital recorders for use during interviews. Careful planning for each project activity will help avoid budget shortfalls. Look to other researchers or experienced budget coordinators to help compile an accurate account of everything needed for the proposed research. Equipment with a cost of over $5,000 has its own budget category.

Many projects require travel as part of the research project or use travel to disseminate results at meetings and conferences. Expenses related to travel must be detailed in the budget, including airfare, hotels, per-diem costs (daily expense rates for travel), and transportation. A realistic average or estimate may be used if exact amounts cannot be calculated (e.g., due to fluctuations in airfares). If the project includes local travel, the PI would include an estimate of miles multiplied by the federal mileage reimbursement rate. Funding agencies and institutions often have travel policies, which must be followed in budget planning.

Expenses not covered in any of the other budget categories are put into an "other" classification. Other expenses might include things like postage, publication costs, incentives, and telephone costs. If uncertain about where to budget project items, look for guidance from the funding agency or seek assistance from a university research office. Most funding agencies allow for some flexibility in spending grant funds, but aiming for an accurate budget is a best practice. Once the project begins, the PI is responsible for reporting how funds are being spent. The funder can require these reports at regular time intervals such as quarterly or annually.

In addition to the itemized and categorized budget, the PI must develop a narrative justification of the budget. The justification describes the responsibilities of key personnel, the reasons for material and supplies requests, and why the travel is needed for the project. The justification must match the proposed budget. An example of a budget justification is depicted in Exhibit 8.2. Once the budget and justification are completed, review the documents carefully to verify the calculations and totals are correct. Grant reviewers do not respond favorably to researchers who submit inaccurate budget proposals.

EXHIBIT 8.2 EXAMPLE OF A GRANT PROPOSAL BUDGET JUSTIFICATION

Personnel (Year 1–5)
Amy A. Eyler, PhD, PI (1.8 academic months, .6 summer months). Dr. Eyler is an assistant professor at the Brown School of Social Work, Program of Public Health. She is a trained behavioral scientist and policy researcher. She has experience in leading effective multicomponent projects related to nutrition, physical activity, and policy. She will be the main investigator for this project and coordinate research team, consultants, and subcontracts. She will also facilitate appropriate dissemination.

Angela Bauer, MD, Coinvestigator (in-kind year 1, 2.4 calendar months year 2–5), Dr. Bauer is board certified in internal medicine with training in endocrinology. She is currently serving as a research fellow in the Division of Endocrinology, Metabolism, and Lipid Research at Washington University School of Medicine. Dr. Bauer will serve as coinvestigator and work closely with Dr. Eyler on project coordination and facilitate the substudy health assessments and analysis.

Rhonda Jones, PhD, MPH, Coinvestigator (.9 academic months, .3 summer months), Dr. Jones is an assistant research professor at the Brown School of Social Work and Prevention Center in St. Louis. She is an epidemiologist with dietetic training. She will assist the project by being the liaison between Morrison staff and the research team and help in dissemination of results.

Jean Harp, PhD, Coinvestigator (.9 academic months, .3 summer months), Dr. Harp is an assistant professor at the Brown School of Social Work, Program of Public Health. He has experience in environmental health and environmental psychology applicable to this project. He will work closely with the research team to analyze geographical aspects of the nutrition environment and assist in all aspects of assessments and data collection.

David Jefferson, PhD, Coinvestigator (.45 academic months, .15 summer months, years 1–2, .9 academic months, .6 summer months year 3–5), Dr. Jefferson is an assistant professor at the Brown School of Social Work, Program of Public Health. He is an economist who has experience in developing appropriate costing and evaluation measures of intervention components. He will work closely with the research team to

(continued)

EXHIBIT 8.2 EXAMPLE OF A GRANT PROPOSAL BUDGET JUSTIFICATION (*continued*)

develop specific criteria needed to produce meaningful economic analysis and assist with the actual cost, feasibility, effectiveness analysis.

Benjamin Young, MPH, Coinvestigator (1.8 calendar months), Mr. Young is a biostatistician with experience in medical and behavioral analysis planning and implementation. He will serve as the data analyst on this project and provide input on the most meaningful way to aggregate and analyze complex data. He will also provide input on dissemination.

TBN, Program Manager (12.0 calendar months), a master's level program manager will be hired to manage the day-to-day activities of the project. This individual will work closely with the project investigators and supervise the other staff on the project. The program manager will also be involved in dissemination activities.

Marcia Abrams, Project Grants Manager (.6 calendar months), will provide support dedicated to the management of the project's budget, including purchasing and procurement, vendor agreements, and maintenance of project budget accounts. She will assist the project manager and the PI with the project goals, procedures for data management and data collection from vendor reports.

TBN, GRA will assist with various tasks related to each aspect of this project. This position is designed for a graduate-level MPH, MSW, or doctoral student enrolled in the WU George Warren Brown School of Social Work. The student will receive a monthly stipend of $900, 24 credits of tuition scholarship annually, and student health insurance. The Brown School of Social Work has a policy in place for graduate research scholars to receive tuition remission and is compliant with the University's "Graduate Research Assistant Tuition Remission" guidelines.

> *Graduate student stipend, $900 × 12 months = $10,800*

Consultants (year 1–5)
None

Supplies (year 1 Only)
One computer ($1,600) with docking station for the Program Manager

Travel
Travel is budgeted for years 2 to 5 of the proposed project. We anticipate two team members attending at least one main public health conference and one main nutrition or food service meeting per year. We budget $1,500 per person to include airfare ($450), hotel ($150/night, three nights = $450), meals and ground transportation ($50/day × 3 days), and conference registration $450.

Other Expenses (year as indicated)
Incentives (year 1, 2, 3). There will be incentives for the 360 participants in the substudy. Individuals will be compensated for their time with $50 at each lab collection plus a

(continued)

EXHIBIT 8.2 EXAMPLE OF A GRANT PROPOSAL BUDGET JUSTIFICATION (*continued*)

bonus of $50 for completing all three screenings (for a total of $200 per participant over the course of the study, Year 3). Additionally, we budgeted $1,125 in year 1 and 3 for U.S. one-dollar coupons as incentive to fill out consumer perception/attitude surveys in cafeterias. For focus groups food service workers, we budgeted $20 for incentives to participate (six groups (2 per cafeteria × 3) with eight participants each) in Year 1 and 3. ($960 in each year).

Lab testing and supplies. The substudy (*n* = 360) will include health screening with lab work 3× (year 1–3). Blood work for HbA1c and cholesterol will be conducted by the Washington University School of Medicine labs at the cost of $50 per test (50 × 3 × 360). An additional cost is estimated at $10.00 for lab supplies (gloves, swabs, needles, bandages, vials, etc.) per person, per test (10 × 3 × 360), years 1 and 2.

Transcription services. We will be conducting interviews (*n* = 5 × 2) and focus groups (*n* = 6 × 2). These will be audiotaped and transcribed to assist with qualitative analysis. This is budgeted at $2,000 for years 2 and 4.

Vendor services. We will contract with Morrison as a vendor ($50K year 1–5) to provide us with monthly sales reporting data, training data, and biannual cafeteria wellness platform assessments. Morrison is the sole food service provider for BJC Cafeterias. This project will involve an evaluation of changes taking place in three of the cafeteria sites (BJC North, BJC South, and SLCH). As a vendor, Morrison will provide reports of cafeteria sales data for the three sites on a monthly basis for each year of the grant. Morrison will also provide additional reports to be collected for the economic benefit analysis. It will also provide menu development and information on the use of price incentives for grill items in each of the cafeterias on a monthly basis. Morrison will provide access to its chefs, retail, and production staff for involvement in this study.

Open-access publication. We aim to publish in an open-access journal,s such as the *Journal of the International Society for Behavioral Nutrition and Physical Activity* to reach a broad academic audience. The approximate cost for an article is $3,000, and we budgeted this for years 4 and 5.

GRA benefits (years 1–5)
> *24 hours of tuition, $1,195/hr = $28,680*
> *Health insurance, $820/year, budget total for year 1 = $29,500*

Indirect Costs
Indirect costs for Washington University in St. Louis are calculated as 52% of direct costs. The year 1 project indirect costs are $277,484 × .52 = $144,292. Years 2–5, respectively: $163,341, $196,661, $147,508, $145,446.

GRA, graduate research assistant; PI, principal investigator; TBN, to be named.

Timelines

Knowing when research activities will occur over the course of the grant project informs budget planning, but also helps to develop the project timeline. Most research grant proposals require a detailed timeline of project activities. The activities should be aligned with the research aims and approach as written in the proposal narrative. Be realistic when planning project activities, as many tasks take longer than expected. If you do not complete your proposed project in the timeframe outlined in the grant, some agencies allow for a no-cost extension. This means the project can continue, but no additional funds will be given toward completion. An example of a project timeline is shown in Exhibit 8.3.

EXHIBIT 8.3 EXAMPLE OF A RESEARCH PROJECT TIMELINE

Aim/Activity	Year 1	Year 2	Year 3	Year 4	Year 5
Aim 1					
Healthy hospital scan	X	X	X	X	X
Wellness platform assessment	X	X	X	X	X
Substudy health assessment	X	X	X		
Food sales assessment	X	X	X	X	
Data analysis	X	X	X	X	X
Aim 2					
Chef interviews	X		X		
Food service focus groups	X		X		
Consumer surveys	X		X		
Data analysis	X	X		X	
Aim 3					
Determine costs			X	X	

(continued)

EXHIBIT 8.3 EXAMPLE OF A RESEARCH PROJECT TIMELINE (*continued*)

Aim/Activity	Year 1		Year 2		Year 3		Year 4		Year 5	
Analysis of sales gains/losses					X		X			
Conduct ROI analysis									X	
Rate strategies by ROI							X		X	
Dissemination plan										
Conduct dissemination										

ROI, return on investment.

CHAPTER DISCUSSION QUESTIONS

1. Compare and contrast the different sources for public health funding. If you wanted to study community access to cardiovascular health screenings, where might you look for funding?
2. What sources could you use to get information on the specific costs of conducting a national survey of hospital administrators on breastfeeding-promotion policies?
3. How might you account for increased costs over the course of a research project in your proposed budget?
4. Why might there be a conflict of interest between a researcher and a funder? How could ethical integrity be maintained and the research be conducted?

RESEARCH PROJECT CHECK-IN

Calculating Costs

Student research projects are good practice for applying new skills, but they probably do not warrant developing a full research budget. Even so, think about how much your study would cost if it were scaled-up. Try to envision the details of what is needed to fully implement a real-world study on the same topic or with the same population as your proposed research. Also think about who might be the best funder for the type of study you are planning. Maybe you could use the student project as a small pilot study, or to gather some formative data to use in a larger study outside of the classroom.

PUBLIC HEALTH RESEARCH METHODS IN REAL LIFE

Show Me (How You Will Spend) The Money!

A well-known foundation just released a notice of fFunding opportunity for exploring adolescent use of vaping devices. Each award maximum is $100,000. The notice described the requirement for projects to focus on students in grades 6 to 8, and that all proposed studies must include qualitative and quantitative data collection. Willa is a doctoral student with an interest in adolescent health. Her advisor is planning to submit a project proposal in response to the foundation announcement, and asked Willa to be a part of it. Willa sees this as an opportunity to get experience in writing grant proposals that she will be able to use as part of her dissertation project.

They plan to interview school administration and other personnel about their perceptions of vaping in five middle schools representing five districts that make up their metropolitan region. They will also conduct two student focus groups at each school. They will use the qualitative data from the focus groups and interviews to develop a tailored electronic survey, which will be distributed to all middle school students within the five school districts.

Willa's advisor asked her to work on the budget. She was to come up with a list of everything they would need to complete the project and estimate costs. She knew from reviewing grant proposals in class that the main categories for research budget were personnel, materials and supplies, travel, and other expenses. She also knew that she had to figure in the university's indirect costs for foundation grants, which was 20% of the total. This meant her total for direct costs would need to total around $83,000. She calculated personnel costs of her advisor's salary, her stipend, and money for another student research assistant. Materials and supplies included recording devices for the focus groups and two digital tablets for the research team to use in the field. She also wanted to include some type of incentive for the students who participated in the focus groups, and maybe a larger incentive drawing for the quantitative survey. After consultation with her middle school-aged sister, she settled on name-brand water bottles at a cost of $30.00 each as the incentive. Students who filled out the survey would be entered into a drawing for five $100.00 online retail gift cards per school. Because the schools were local and easily reached with public transportation, no travel funds were needed. Willa added costs for a professional transcriptionist to expedite qualitative analysis. The university had a subscription to online survey software so there was no budget item for that.

When she added everything up, she was shocked to find she was over budget by $20,000! She needed to go over and prioritize spending. The largest expense was personnel at $58,000. Salaries and fringe benefits took up a lot of the budget. There was really no way to lower that. She contemplated taking out the research assistant, but this project was going to be a lot of work and they would need extra help as neither Willa nor her advisor would be full time on this project. She decided to take out the digital recorders and the tablets. She worked at a research center with other investigators and she confirmed she could borrow these rather than purchase them. She also decided to reduce the incentives to a $10 gift card per focus group participant and a drawing for one gift card per school. Professional transcription was an absolute necessity. The transcription agency she listed in the budget had a reduced rate for the university and had a reputation for fast and accurate work. There would be no additional reductions there.

Finally, after several iterations, Willa had a budget that totaled $82,678. She discussed the final proposed budget with her advisor and was lauded for her expert budgeting efforts. Willa just hoped that she did not forget something!

Critical Thinking Questions

1. How would you go about planning for a research budget differently than Willa did?
2. What things might Willa have included in the budget that she did not?
3. How would else could Willa have revised the budget to fit within the $100,000 maximum? What else could she have cut?
4. How would you budget for incentives with this age group? What do you think it would take to get adolescents to participate in focus groups?
5. Fortunately, Willa had some budgeting experience before this proposal. How might you get some budget training if you were asked to prepare a research budget as a complete novice?

COUNCIL ON EDUCATION FOR PUBLIC HEALTH FOUNDATIONAL KNOWLEDGE AND COMPETENCIES

Foundational Knowledge
Profession and Science of Public Health
- Explain the critical importance of evidence in advancing public health knowledge.

Foundational Competencies
Planning and Management to Promote Health
- Explain the basic principles and tools of budget and resource management.
- Select methods to evaluate public health programs.

REFERENCES

1. Centers for Disease Control and Prevention. Ten great public health achievements — United States, 1900–1999. *MMWR*. 1999;48(12):241-243. Accessed January 27, 2019. https://www.cdc.gov/mmwr/preview/mmwrhtml/00056796.htm

2. Lauer M. NIH annual snapshot – FY 2018 by the numbers | NIH extramural nexus. 2019. Accessed September 19, 2019. https://nexus.od.nih.gov/all/2019/03/13/nih-annual-snapshot-fy-2018-by-the-numbers

3. Fineberg HV. The paradox of disease prevention. *JAMA*. 2013;310(1):85. doi:10.1001/jama.2013.7518

4. Council on Education for Public Health. Accreditation criteria for schools of public health and programs of public health. 2016. Accessed September 19, 2019. https://media.ceph.org/documents/2016.Criteria.pdf

5. Viergever RF, Hendriks TCC. The 10 largest public and philanthropic funders of health research in the world: what they fund and how they distribute their funds. *Health Res Policy Syst*. 2016;14(1):12. doi:10.1186/s12961-015-0074-z

6. World Health Organization. Research. Accessed September 19, 2019. *WHO*. 2018. https://www.who.int/topics/research/en

7. National Institutes of Health. NIH research portfolio online reporting tools (RePORT). 2019. Accessed September 17, 2019. https://report.nih.gov

8. Moses H, Matheson DHM, Cairns-Smith S, et al. The anatomy of medical research. *JAMA*. 2015;313(2):174. doi:10.1001/jama.2014.15939

9. US Department of Health and Human Services. Prevention and Public Health Fund. 2018. Accessed September 17, 2019. https://www.hhs.gov/open/prevention/index.html

10. Centers for Disease Control and Prevention. Congressional justifications budget 2019. 2019. Accessed September 17, 2019. https://www.cdc.gov/budget/fy2019/congressional-justification.html

11. National Council of Nonprofits. What is a "nonprofit"? National Council of Nonprofits. 2019. Accessed September 19, 2019. https://www.councilofnonprofits.org/what-is-a-nonprofit

12. Statista. Number of foundations in the U.S. 2015. 2019. Accessed September 17, 2019. https://www.statista.com/statistics/250878/number-of-foundations-in-the-united-states

13. Maani Hessari N, Ruskin G, McKee M, et al. Public meets private: conversations between Coca Cola and the CDC. *Milbank Q*. 2019;97(1):74-90. doi:10.1111/1468-0009.12368

14. Robert Wood Johnson Foundation. Budget preparation guidelines. 2019. Accessed September 18, 2019. https://anr.rwjf.org/templates/external/BPG_Standard.pdf

15. Bill and Melinda Gates Foundation. Indirect cost policy. 2017. Accessed September 18, 2019. https://docs.gatesfoundation.org/documents/indirect_cost_policy.pdf

16. Olinger D. CU nutrition expert accepts $550,000 from Coca-Cola for obesity campaign. *The Denver Post*. December 26, 2015. Accessed September 18, 2019. https://www.denverpost.com/2015/12/26/cu-nutrition-expert-accepts-550000-from-coca-cola-for-obesity-campaign

17. O'Connor A. Coca-Cola funds scientists who shift blame for obesity away from bad diets. *New York Times Well Blogs*. August 9, 2015. Accessed September 18, 2019. https://well.blogs.nytimes.com/2015/08/09/coca-cola-funds-scientists-who-shift-blame-for-obesity-away-from-bad-diets

ADDITIONAL READINGS AND RESOURCES

Fabbri A, Lai A, Grundy Q, et al. The influence of industry sponsorship on the research agenda: a scoping review. *Am J Public Health*. 2018;108(11):e9–e16. doi:10.2105/AJPH.2018.304677

Candid. Foundation directory online. 2019. Accessed September 18, 2019. https://fdo.foundationcenter.org

III

QUANTITATIVE RESEARCH

This section describes ways to conduct research using quantitative or numeric data. Chapter 9, Quantitative Data Collection, outlines common ways to collect quantitative data, such as surveys and through systematic observation. Technological advancements have certainly increased the ways data can be collected. Online surveys, text message data collection, and webcam observations are evolving as effective methods for quantitative research. This chapter also describes best practices for developing good survey questions. Chapter 10, Quantitative Data Analysis, outlines the next step in a quantitative research study—data analysis. Sections on recoding data variables and issues, such as missing data, provide useful best practices. This chapter also includes information on descriptive statistics, inferential statistics, and some basic-level parametric and nonparametric testing. Bundled with information from the previous chapters, this section guides the researcher through the steps needed for quality quantitative research.

Quantitative Data Collection

The sample survey has been transformed from being a comfortable face-to-face conversation to a highly impersonal experience that with increasing frequency is mediated by an electronic device.

—Don Dillman, PhD, survey expert

LEARNING OBJECTIVES

After reading this chapter, the reader will be able to

- Compare and contrast ways to collect quantitative data.
- Develop quality survey questions.
- Define and provide examples of objective measurements in public health research.
- Understand the influence of technology on quantitative data collection.

INTRODUCTION

We have come a long way from face-to-face data collection and paper-and-pencil surveys as the only choices for gathering research information. Today, there are many data-source options, and with technology quickly advancing, more options are constantly emerging. What data source or sources are best for your quantitative research study? As all methods of data collection have strengths and weaknesses, the best choice depends on several factors. First, refer to your research question and hypothesis. What do you need to know? The specific information necessary to answer your research question and/or test your hypothesis may limit your data-source choices. You will need to consider the importance of gathering objective data (e.g., accelerometry, which measures physical activity) versus self-reported data (e.g., survey) in achieving your research objective. See Exhibit 9.1 for more information on objectively measured versus self-reported data sources. Second, consider your topic. There may be unique advantages and disadvantages to data sources for research on sensitive topics or topics prone to social desirability bias. For example, an anonymous online survey about sexual behavior may be a better choice than an in-person survey. There are other factors that may influence choice of data collection relating to the research process itself. Consider the accessibility of the data. Is the source readily available? Is it feasible to gather the data within the timeline of your project? What are the expenses associated with your data-source options? There are costs associated with implementing a survey, but there also may be costs in accessing existing data or documents. Remember to keep in mind how you intend to analyze the data. An online survey platform allows for quick and easy ways to export data for analysis. Paper survey data have to be manually entered into a database, and due to the potential for human error, this method often requires resources for double data entry. In addition, the time and complexity of preparing data for the analysis phase needs to be considered along with your data-source options.

EXHIBIT 9.1 SELF-REPORT VERSUS OBJECTIVE MEASUREMENT

Although commonly used in public health research, there are several limitations to using self-reported data. First, the data may be an inaccurate reflection of the actual behavior, symptom, attitude, and so on. Sometimes the inaccuracies are due to social desirability bias. People may not want to report truthfully about sensitive topics or topics for which they may feel judged by the way they respond. Other times the inaccuracies may be due to misunderstanding what is being asked. Questions worded in a confusing way, or that are not consistent with the literacy or culture of the respondents, can distort the level of truth in the data. Recall is another common limitation in self-reports. Remembering past behaviors, actions, or attitudes may be challenging. Can you remember what you had for dinner yesterday?

One way to overcome some of the limitations of self-report is to use objective measures when possible. Objective data is collected or obtained through verifiable procedures or strategies. For example, instead of asking people to report their blood pressure, you would actually measure it at the time of data collection. Several studies have compared the accuracy of self-reported data to data obtained from objective measures. Mosca et al. assessed the prevalence rates of hypertension and hypercholesterolemia from healthcare provider measurements to self-reports of these two conditions. The prevalence for both were significantly higher when measured objectively (hypertension = 64%; hypercholesterolemia = 72.1%) as compared to self-reports (hypertension = 37%; hypercholesterolemia = 41.1%).[1] Conversely, people tend to over-report certain behavior such as physical activity. In general, about 50% of Americans report achieving the recommended amounts of physical activity.[2] However, when compared to objectively assessed physical movement via accelerometer, only about 8% of Americans actually achieve the recommended amounts of physical activity.[3] Discrepancies have also been found in comparisons between perceived and objective measures of access to neighborhood resources. Sometimes people are not aware of their proximity to parks or grocery stores in their community, or if these destinations even exist.[4] Matching self-reported data to geographic information system (GIS) maps and other novel mapping techniques has helped improve the accuracy of environmental measures. Although self-reported data may be an easy data source, triangulating it with objective measures may strengthen your study.

QUANTITATIVE DATA COLLECTION

Self-Reports. Self-reported data is an individual's own account of factors such as attitudes, symptoms, beliefs, or behaviors. This type of data is relatively easy to gather through surveys or interviews, and is commonly used in public health research. Interviews and qualitative data collection are discussed in Chapter 12, Qualitative Data Collection. For many public health topics, reliable and valid surveys or questionnaires already exist. Using existing scales saves the time and effort of developing a measurement tool from scratch, and particularly strengthens your study if the tools have statistics to support their reliability and validity.

Whether you are asking people for information through surveys or interviews, well-written questions are vital to reducing systematic error. There are several common mistakes to avoid. Questions may be phrased in a way that "leads" the respondent to answer in a particular way. "Should effective parenting include prohibiting screen time?" The word "effective" can promote a different response than if more neutral wording was used. Remove judgment-based words from questions. Double-barreled questions can also cause confusion for the respondent. Sometimes researchers will "double-up" on the topics within a single question. Consider the question "Do you support the use of public funds for a new park and a tax increase as a source of those funds?" Perhaps the respondent supports public funding for parks, but does not support a tax increase. Never put more than one concept in the same question. Some double-barreled questions may not be so obvious. Suppose you ask children in your study to state their level of agreement with the statement "My parents exercise with me." What if the respondent is from a single-parent family or is being raised by adults other than parents? What if their mother exercises with them, but not their father? They will not be able to answer this question accurately. Carefully consider the wording when developing questions. Ambiguous terms should also be avoided. In the question, "How often do you eat meat?" what is meant by "often"? What is meant by "meat"? Giving respondents more precise definitions will invoke more accurate responses. A better question would be: "On average, how frequently do you eat red meat? Include beef or lamb, all steaks, chops, and roasts. Do not include pork or chicken." Response options would include a fill-in-the-blank section for times per day, times per week, or times per month. This question not only defines what is meant by "meat," but also provides an opportunity for the respondent to record their frequency in a way most meaningful to their behavior. If you asked, "How many times per week do you eat red meat?", the respondent might not be able to provide a relevant response if they eat it once a month. Pilot-testing your questions with members of the population you wish to survey will help avoid some of these mistakes. **Cognitive response testing** is another way to gain insight into how respondents may perceive questions. Cognitive response testing involves an in-depth interview with a small number of respondents who are similar to the target survey population. Researchers using this method of pretesting ask the cognitive response testing participants for details on how they interpret the questions, whether the concepts make sense, and what factors determined their answers. Data from cognitive response testing can inform revisions needed, thus reducing the chance of measurement error. The content of the responses in cognitive response testing is less relevant than the participant's perception of the question.

Questions can be open ended or closed ended. **Open-ended questions** are worded in such a way that the respondent can answer in phrases or sentences. These questions elicit a broad and unique set of responses. Open-ended questions are also helpful when researching new topics or ideas. However, open-ended questions can be more time-consuming to use for the researcher. Information from responses has to be categorized or coded in order to analyze it quantitatively.

EXAMPLE: Describe the commute from your home to your place of employment.

I ride my bike a few minutes to the bus stop from my house. Then I catch the #9, usually at 7:55. I get off the bus and ride about 10 minutes to my building. I clock in at 9:00, but sometimes I am late.

Responses to this question may fall into categories of mode and time. Pilot-testing open-ended questions can be informative to the researcher. The answers to open-ended questions may provide data used to develop more precise questions. Maybe you never considered asking about multiple ways a person commutes to work. If this information is helpful to answering your research question, you might add more specific instructions about describing all modes of commuting.

Closed-ended questions are those for which response options are provided. Data from closed-ended questions are typically easier to analyze than open-ended data because the response categories can easily be converted into numeric codes for quantitative analysis. However, the response options may not be exhaustive or limited to unique responses. Many closed-ended questions allow respondents to choose more than one answer or add in their response if it is not an option (such as "Other"—*fill in the blank*).

EXAMPLE: On a typical day, how do you commute to work? (Check all that apply)
- ○ Walk
- ○ Bicycle
- ○ Bus or other public transportation
- ○ Single-occupancy vehicle
- ○ Carpool
- ○ Electric scooter

Other: _____ (please indicate other options)

Whatever type of questions you choose for your self-reported data source, remember, good questions are

- specifically related to your research question;
- brief, clear, and concise;
- neutral, nonbiased;
- inquiries about a single concept; and
- aligned with respondent's literacy and culture.

HOW DO YOU GET PEOPLE TO PROVIDE DATA?

Getting people to people provide their data can sometimes be challenging. Today, people are inundated with requests for information. Go to any retail store, and chances are your receipt shows an opportunity to get some sort of coupon if you fill out a satisfaction survey. Every day, our email inboxes are filled with requests for a "few minutes of our time to fill

CULTURALLY COMPETENT DATA COLLECTION

As discussed in Chapter 3, Ethics in Public Health Research, public health researchers should incorporate cultural competence into all steps of the research process. The national culturally and linguistically appropriate services standards (CLAS) are relevant to operationalization and measurement. The principal standard of CLAS is "Provide effective, equitable, understandable, and respectful quality care and services that are responsive to diverse cultural health beliefs and practices, preferred languages, health literacy, and other communication needs."[25] Think of measurement and data collection as "services." When developing definitions for your variables or ways to measure them, always keep the unique needs and characteristics of the target population in mind. Two ways to ensure appropriate measures are to (a) include input from members of the target population when you develop measures, and (b) pilot test the measures with a sample of the target population. Conducting culturally competent research studies will advance healthy equity and improve health disparities.

out a brief survey." When using many websites, a box will appear asking questions about the usefulness of the information on the webpage. How can researchers compete for survey responses? According to Don A. Dillman,[5] an expert in survey methodology, the theory of social exchange is useful in motivating people to respond. In this theory, three key issues need to be addressed. Each issue is explored in the following text.

How can the perceived rewards (benefits) for responding be increased? Suggestions for increasing the rewards or benefits include the following:

- Provide information about the survey and how results will be used to benefit participants or the population.
- Aski for help or assistance. People may feel a sense of reward for helping.
- Support group values by making the connection from the survey to the target respondent group.
- Give tangible rewards. Appropriate and timely incentives given in exchange for survey burden may increase perceived benefit. Look to past research, pilot testing, or stakeholder input to determine the most relevant incentive.
- Inform people that opportunities to respond are limited. This may increase the perceived value of responding.

How can the perceived costs of responding be reduced? Suggestions for decreasing the costs of responding include the following:

- Make it convenient to respond. Many web-based survey platforms now offer mobile-friendly options so people can conveniently respond to a survey using their cell phones.
- Make the questionnaire short. Consider including only questions essential to your research focus.
- Minimize requests for sensitive information, and, if needed, emphasize confidentiality or anonymity in responses.
- Include a way to save survey responses, in case they want to return to the survey at a later time.

How can trust be established so that people believe the rewards will outweigh the costs of responding? Suggestions for increasing trust include the following:

- Obtain sponsorship from a legitimate authority. Carefully consider history and perceived trust between academic institutions and community when determining sponsorship.
- Ensure the confidentiality of the information being collected. Institutional review board certification with contact information can help boost faith in confidentiality.
- Identify the request for information as important to some outcome relevant to the respondent or population group.

Using these best practices may get people to respond to a survey, but how do you know you have enough data, or whether the group of people who responded are representative of your target population? Calculating the response rate is the first step. Simply stated, the **response rate** is the number of people who completed your survey divided by the number in the sample population. For example, if you send your survey to 500 people and 250 respond to it, your response rate is 50%. Calculating response rates is not as simple as it seems. You need to factor in the number of nonworking telephone numbers for phone surveys, return-to-sender postal surveys, or email bounce backs to calculate the most accurate response rate. Acceptable response rates vary by mode of survey, discipline, and topic. Look to the literature on your topic of study to investigate average response rates.

Another way of identifying the representativeness of your respondents is to compare demographics with the larger sample. For example, if you know the racial/ethnic breakdown of a community you are surveying and you ask a race/ethnicity question on your survey, you can compare your survey sample with the greater community to justify representation. If the sample of respondents is significantly different from the larger population, results are less likely to be generalizable to the group.

RACE AND ETHNICITY

Simply stated, race is associated with biology, and ethnicity is associated with culture within a geographical region. In 2010, the U.S. Census assessed these two concepts in separate questions. The question on race reflected a self-identification and social definition of race, but was not intended to define race biologically, anthropologically, or genetically. Ethnicity assessment included self-identification of Latinx, Hispanic, or Spanish origin. In addition to choosing ethnicity, census respondents could also select a race category. A person could respond as White <u>and</u> of Hispanic origin. Research and public comment about the inaccuracy of this method was implemented. Although there has been movement to improve the way the census race and ethnicity questions are asked, the 2020 Census included the same separate questions previously used in 2010. Accurate assessment of demographics is vital to making policy decisions on racial disparities in health and environmental risks. The topic of race and ethnicity will likely be revisited for the 2030 Census.

Source: U.S. Census Bureau. About: Race. 2018. Accessed September 6, 2020. https://www.census.gov/topics/population/race/about.html

METHODS OF SURVEY IMPLEMENTATION

Telephone surveys are one way to gather public health data. The Behavioral Risk Factor Surveillance System (BRFSS) is one of the largest telephone survey systems in the United States. BRFSS is used by the Centers for Disease Control and Prevention (CDC) for health-related telephone surveys, and collects data from more than 400,000 adult interviews each year.[6] The BRFSS sets a standard for telephone data-collection methodology, which can be used in other research studies. Simply stated, methods include randomly selecting phone numbers, then calling to collect responses from people with those numbers. However, telephone data collection is becoming obsolete for many reasons. In 2018, more than half of American homes had only wireless telephones.[7] In the past, landline phone numbers had area codes associated with specific geographic regions, making it easy to match data with community and U.S. Census data. The area codes on cell phone numbers may not match the geographic region of the user. Previously, the area code 216 matched the phone numbers of people living in the Cleveland, Ohio, region. Today, a person who got a cell while living in Cleveland who moved to another state and kept the original cell-phone number, still has a 216 area code. If you are interested in information related specifically to the Cleveland region and randomly select phone numbers with the area code 216, you may not produce the best sample. Also, people are becoming less likely to answer a call from an unfamiliar number, making gathering data more challenging. A 2019 analysis of cellular call data showed 52% of all calls went unanswered.[8] This is not of benefit to researchers trying to collect data by telephone. In a survey on perception of physical activity policy, it took calls to 10,440 cellular customers to get data from 79 respondents![9] The amount of time and resources needed to collect data in this way should be carefully considered when planning a research study.

Mailing paper copies of surveys to the target population is also a way to collect survey data. As in the case of telephone data, this method has advantages and disadvantages. Address lists are fairly easy to access, and the physical addresses help limit respondents to specific geographic areas of interest. However, printing, paper, postage, and return postage can be costly. Many researchers using mail surveys also send out reminders to fill out the survey after the original request was sent. The cost of the reminders (printing and postage) also needs to be factored into the budget. Time is a budget item, too. Transferring data from the hard copies into databases needs human resources, and can be time-consuming. Even though it may be easy to access addresses, people may move or homes may be vacant. Undeliverable surveys are "returned to sender" by the postal service. This can pose challenges to calculating response rates and getting accurate representation of the target population. Lastly, the use of the U.S. Postal Service for first-class mail has steadily declined over the past 5 years.[10] The culture shift to using online services may impact the effectiveness of collecting data through mail surveys, especially for certain age groups. In 2018, the U.S. Inspector General's Office conducted a survey to gain perspective on Millennials and the mail. Results showed respondents in the 18-to-34 age group were much less likely than older age groups to check their mailbox frequently, and much more likely to pay bills online rather than through the mail.[11] These trends should be considered when choosing survey methods.

Telephone and mail surveys are still used in public health research, but changes in technology and population preferences are causing a shift in data-collection methodology. The Internet provides one of the latest venues for collecting data in public health research. Surveys can be implemented through email, websites, or social media. Target audiences for these surveys can be broad and unrestricted, or more narrowly focused. Online surveys may be targeted to email lists or specific interest groups through, for example, focused social media pages. One example of a targeted online method is panel research. In **panel research**, online survey companies merge commercial lists of potential respondents to develop a sample frame, which can then be narrowed to match characteristics of the target research population (e.g., women age 50–65 years). These frames can be useful if the research study includes multiple data collection from the same people. The Health and Retirement Study is an example of panel research. The sample consists of 20,000 Americans over the age of 50, and the study collects data every 2 years on topics such as income, work, health, and healthcare.[12] Targeted panel lists are convenient if purchased through an online survey company, but can be costly. The more specific the population or the more difficult it is to reach the population, the more effort and resources will be needed to collect the data. For example, data from men and women aged 18 to 22 who live in urban areas will be easier to access than that of older adults who are primary caregivers of grandchildren and who are living in a specific region or community.

There are several advantages to using online surveys to collect data compared with paper-and-pencil surveys. First, the internet allows for broad reach. In 2019, about 90% of Americans reported using the internet.[13] Although this percentage varies by demographic group, online access is almost ubiquitous. Online surveys allow for more complex survey design than in mailed surveys. If all questions may not apply to all respondents, online surveys may provide skip patterns (i.e., where only the relevant questions show up on the screen) making them less cumbersome than printed surveys. Suppose you ask a question about smoking status. With an online survey, only respondents who smoke would get a set of questions about history and frequency of smoking. These questions would not be relevant from those who do not smoke, so they would not have to view or skip them.

Online surveys can also incorporate graphics, pictures, colors, and interactive question formats (Exhibit 9.2). Pop-up definitions of terms can be used to improve clarity and understandability (Exhibit 9.3). Many online survey platforms allow for mobile phone responses, too. Another advantage is the ease with which online survey response data can be transferred into statistical analysis software. This eliminates the step of inputting data by hand from hard-copy surveys. Online surveys can be a cost-effective way of collecting data, as it requires no printing or postage. With the increasing cost of postage, using online versus mailed surveys can reduce a research budget.

Online surveys do have some disadvantages. Certain populations (e.g., older adults) may be more difficult to reach using this method. In addition, online survey invitations could be ignored or deleted due to the number of requests people receive. Fraudulent responses may also be a concern. It is easy to click through and respond to a survey without actually reading the questions. Your research question and study design parameters should inform the best survey method for your study. It may even be appropriate to use a combination of methods in order to meet your data-collection needs. Table 9.1 summarizes the advantages and disadvantages of survey implementation methods.

EXHIBIT 9.2 EXAMPLES OF ONLINE QUESTION FORMATS

Example 1. Tab slide

To what extent does your workspace enhance or interfere with your individual work effectiveness?

ENHANCES   **INTERFERES**

Slide tab to answer

Example 2. Graphic

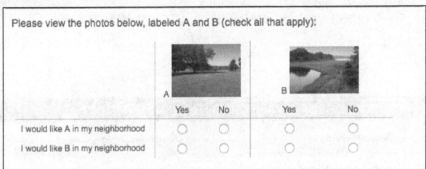

Please view the photos below, labeled A and B (check all that apply):

	Yes	No	Yes	No
I would like A in my neighborhood	○	○	○	○
I would like B in my neighborhood	○	○	○	○

Example 3. Map

Please click once on the map in the city block or general area of where you live (your answer will appear in green, with a check mark in the middle).

Please click twice on the map on the outdoor space you use most frequently (your answer will appear in red, with an x in the middle).

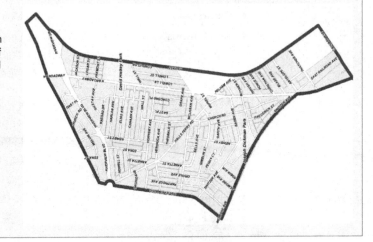

EXHIBIT 9.3 EXAMPLE OF A POP-UP/ROLLOVER DEFINITION IN AN ONLINE SURVEY

Where do you live?

I live on campus

I live in off-campus university housing

I live off-campus in non-university housing

My housing situation is unstable   **Transient, intermittent (e.g. couch surfing)**

TABLE 9.1 COMPARISON OF SURVEY IMPLEMENTATION METHODS

Survey Type	Advantages	Disadvantages
Mail	• Geographic targets • Easy to develop • Broad reach • Anonymous	• Data input • Returned surveys • Cost of postage • Limits formats (e.g., complex skip patterns) • Generational differences
Telephone	• Allows for clarification • More personal approach • No visual aids • Can screen for demographics	• Changing social norms around phone use • Difficult to target geographic region
Online	• Large distribution • Low cost • Allows complex format • Database formed • Respondents can answer in private	• Nonresponse • Not equally accessible • Bounce-backs • Do not know who is actually completing the survey • Lower response rate

TEXTING WHILE SURVEYING

According to the Gallup Corporation, a leader in analytics, almost 75% of American adults with cellphones report checking their phone at least once an hour.[24] The growth in popularity of texting as a form of communication makes this a potential way to contact survey participants. Smartphone apps are available to facilitate delivery and data from texting surveys. Although promising as a research data-collection method, there are some limitations to this method of survey administration. Questions need to be brief (i.e., 160 characters) and surveys cannot be too long or complex. Some demographics have lower cellphone and smartphone ownership, and some groups (such as older adults) might be less likely to participate. Also, regulations require consent to receive text-message surveys. Gallup has conducted several pilot tests using different forms of text-messaging surveys, and they do not recommend conducting stand-alone text- message surveys for the general population.[24] However, technology and culture shifts can impact the acceptance and use of texting as a surveying method. Keep an eye on the literature within your topic and population of interest and data from national survey firms (such as Gallup) to get the latest advice for best practices.

OBJECTIVE MEASUREMENT

Objective measurements reduce the bias from the subjectivity inherent in self-reported data. You can ask people to report how much they weigh, or you could weigh them on an accurate scale. The scale provides an objective measurement of a person's weight, whereas the self-reported weight may be a subjective assessment, a guess, or an inaccurate reflection of their true weight. Objective measures improve the rigor in public health research.

Technology is enhancing the ability to accurately capture data. For example, people in research studies can wear small devices that track their physical activity and exact geographic location of that activity. Researchers download the data from the devices and get an accurate measure of how active people were and where those activities took place. Mobile phones can also facilitate objective data collection. For example, rather than having to recall food intake, people in nutrition studies can take pictures of their meals with their cell-phone cameras. Image classification technology can be used to process the pictures and classify food items. Mobile phone and computer apps can measure blood pressure, heart rate, sleep quality, and many other concepts relevant to public health research. The technology develops quickly and evidence on validity and reliability may still be emerging. Look to the literature for documentation of the best objective measurement for the study topic.

Observations are another way of collecting objective data. Researchers can observe people, places, or situations directly. For example, rather than relying on self-reports of neighborhood resources available, a researcher can visit a community and record the quantity and quality of those resources. See Exhibit 9.4 for a template for recording observations of hand hygiene in healthcare settings. Observations can also complement other data-collection methods. You could survey people to get their perceptions of the community resources and

EXHIBIT 9.4 AMBULATORY SURGICAL CENTER INFECTION CONTROL SURVEYOR WORKSHEET: HAND HYGIENE

INFECTION CONTROL AND RELATED PRACTICES

INSTRUCTIONS

- Please **select ONE bubble** for each "Was Practice Performed?" question, unless otherwise noted.
- If N/A *or unable to observe is selected as the* response, please explain why there is no associated observation, or why the question is not applicable, in the *surveyor notes* box. *Surveyors should attempt to assess the practice by interview or document review if unable to observe the actual practice during survey.*
- *During the survey, observations or concerns may prompt the surveyor to request and review specific policies and procedures. Surveyors are expected to use their judgment and review only those documents necessary to investigate their concern(s) or validate their observations.*

I.   Hand Hygiene

Observations are to focus on staff directly involved in patient care (e.g., physicians, nurses, CRNAs).

Hand hygiene should be observed not only during the case being followed, but also while making other observations in the ASC throughout the survey.

Unless otherwise indicated, a **NO** response to any question **must** be cited as a deficient practice in relation to 42 CFR 416.51 (a).

Practices to Be Assessed	Was Practice Performed?	Surveyor Notes:
A. All patient care areas have items *readily accessible, in appropriate locations:*		
a. Soap and water	○ Yes ○ **No**	
b. Alcohol-based hand rubs	○ Yes ○ **No**	
i. If alcohol-based hand rub is available in patient care areas, it is installed as required. **(There are LSC requirements at 42 CFR 416.44(b)(5)for installation of alcohol-based hand rubs.)**	○ Yes ○ **No**	

(continued)

EXHIBIT 9.4 AMBULATORY SURGICAL CENTER INFECTION CONTROL SURVEYOR WORKSHEET: HAND HYGIENE (*continued*)

INFECTION CONTROL AND RELATED PRACTICES

B. Staff perform hand hygiene:

    a. After removing gloves

        ○ Yes

        ○ **No**

    b. Before direct patient contact

        ○ yes

        ○ **No**

    c. After direct patient contact

        ○ Yes

        ○ **No**

    d. Before performing invasive procedures (e.g., placing an IV)

        ○ Yes

        ○ **No**

        ○ *Unable to observe*

    e. After contact with blood, bodily fluids, or contaminated surfaces (even if gloves are worn)

        ○ Yes

        ○ **No**

        ○ *Unable to observe*

C. Regarding gloves, staff:

    a. Wear gloves for procedures that might involve contact with blood or bodily fluids

        ○ Yes

        ○ **No**

        ○ *Unable to observe*

    b. Wear gloves when handling potentially contaminated patient equipment

        ○ Yes

        ○ **No**

        ○ *Unable to observe*

(continued)

EXHIBIT 9.4 AMBULATORY SURGICAL CENTER INFECTION CONTROL SURVEYOR WORKSHEET: HAND HYGIENE (continued)

INFECTION CONTROL AND RELATED PRACTICES

c. Remove gloves before moving to the next tasks and/or patient

○ Yes

○ **No**

○ *Unable to observe*

D. Personnel providing direct patient care do not wear artificial fingernails and/or extensions when in direct contact with patients.

ASC, ambulatory surgery center; CFR, care facilities requirement; CRNA, certified registered nurse anesthetist; IV, intravenous; LSC, Life Safety Code.

Source: Centers for Medicare and Medicaid Services. Ambulatory Surgical Center (ACS) Infection Control Surveyor Worksheet. n.d. Accessed September 22, 2019. https://www.cms.gov/Regulations-and-Guidance/Guidance/Manuals/downloads/som107_exhibit_351.pdf[14]

compare these with direct-observation data. The combination of both types of information can provide a broad perspective of the issue.

Systematic observation is a way to ensure accuracy in reporting what is observed. Developing a "system" or structure for methodical observation reduces the chance of observer bias. Tested and validated systematic protocols already exist for many public health research topics. For use in physical activity research, the System for Observing Play and Recreation in Communities (SOPARC) is a validated direct-observation tool for assessing parks and recreation areas.[15] Wide acceptance of this research tool resulted in other adaptations such as System for Observing Play and Leisure Activity in Youth (SOPLAY)[16] and System for Observing Fitness Instruction Time (SOFIT).[17] The Nutrition Environment Measures Survey (NEMS) provides measures and protocols for systematic observations of food vending, grocery stores, and restaurants.[18] Look to the literature on your research topic to identify existing observation tools. If the information is not accessible, request a copy from the corresponding author. Most often, researchers are thrilled that someone is interested in their study. This will save you from developing one from scratch and promote validity and reliability of data collection.

Although objective measurement can be the "gold standard" of data collection, it may not be feasible for all research studies. Weighing people in person improves accuracy of the data, but it also takes time, personnel, and space. This may not be possible for large, multisite studies, or studies with limited budgets. Traveling to many places for systematic observation might also be a challenge. For studies incorporating observation of spaces, researchers may be able to use technology to reduce observation burden. Publicly available web-based cameras (e.g., traffic cameras or cameras used to identify weather patterns) capture images that can be used for many different types of public health research. The

Archive of Many Outdoor Scenes (AMOS) is a database of compiled images from over 20,000 publicly available webcams throughout the world.[19] Researchers analyzed a sample of AMOS images to identify how changes in street intersections impact transportation in those spaces.[20] Crowdsourcing is another way to reduce observation burden through technology. **Crowdsourcing** uses input and data from a large number of people with the help of technology. This method is growing in popularity in public health surveillance and has been used in the areas of tobacco control, physical activity, and environmental health.[21] In one study, Moorhead et al. used crowdsourcing to test the feasibility of a smartphone app to estimate calories of food using a photo.[26] Researchers are also using crowdsourcing from online reviews of restaurants to identify incidence of food-borne illness in restaurants.[22, 23] Because crowdsourcing is an emerging way to collect data, more evidence is needed on the rigor and validity of its use.

AVAILABLE RECORDS

Primary data collection is not a requirement for public health research. Many types of data and records already exist, and they could be incorporated into your research design. **Secondary data,** data already collected for surveillance or from a previous study, is a viable option for exploring many public health topics. The U.S. Census and the CDC's BRFSS are two common public health data sources.

There are many other sources of existing information for use in public health research. If you are interested in policy research, there are municipal, state, and federal policy databases available for investigaion. Governmental agencies collect different types of data and make them available for public use. For example, the U.S. Environmental Protection Agency provides public access to Air Quality System (AQS) data (www.epa.gov/aqs). The National Center for Education Statistics (NCES) collects data on schools and universities (nces.ed.gov/datatools). Advocacy agencies can also be a source for available records. AmericaWalks tracks state and local initiatives to create walkable communities (americawalks.org). Media of all types are archived, and can be used as data for quantitative and qualitative analysis. Many existing records are easily accessible through the Internet, but developing and documenting comprehensive search strategies will ensure representation of the resources you use.

CHAPTER DISCUSSION QUESTIONS

1. What factors should influence choice of data collection in a public health research study?
2. How might you ensure the survey questions are relevant to your target population?
3. Describe ways you could collect quantitative data on the topic of safety equipment use in community sport programs?
4. How are technological advancements changing data-collection methods? What are the benefits and disadvantages of using these methods for public health research?

RESEARCH PROJECT CHECK-IN

"I'd Like to Ask You Some Questions."

If you are planning to do a quantitative study, you will need a means of collecting and compiling numeric data. How will you get this information? Look to the literature to see whether surveys exist. Even if the actual survey or step–by-step methodology is not presented in the articles, you can email the authors to request this information. Most are happy to share their information. A lot of effort goes into a research project, and you want to make sure to get the best outcome possible, so once you develop your questions or other methods of gathering data, be sure to pilot test them. A glitch in data collection can really mess things up, and pilot testing is like glitch prevention.

PUBLIC HEALTH RESEARCH METHODS IN REAL LIFE

The Ask

You cannot do analysis without data, and this was what was troubling to Vanetta and her research team. Vanetta was leading a project to identify the extent to which neighborhood residents knew how to protect themselves from mosquito-borne illnesses. The local public health department found mosquitos carrying the West Nile virus concentrated in one suburban area of the county, and were starting to see cases of illness in this region. To help in these efforts, Vanetta developed a yard and neighborhood audit tool for residents to use to collect data and serve as "citizen scientists." She learned of this method at an environmental health conference, and colleagues from another state reported its effectiveness. Results also showed that by having residents involved in this way, the tool was also useful in increasing awareness of ways to protect against these types of illnesses.

Vanetta's team distributed surveys to the mailboxes of all the residents in the neighborhood of interest. The survey included a series of questions about yard conditions and preventive measures. One component of the survey was a checklist of items prone to standing water, a known breeding ground for mosquitos. The question was, "Please check all of the items that currently exist on your property." The list included potholes, blocked gutters, birdbaths, old tires, containers, and flowerpots. If standing water was an issue, Vanetta's plan was to implement an intervention to educate residents on ways to improve mosquito prevention.

Two weeks after delivering the survey, only 10 of the 100 residents had responded. Not one indicated any standing water existed on their property. Vanetta was concerned about the low response rate, but also concerned about the data. Her encounters in this neighborhood led her to believe most yards had at least one item common for holding standing water. After consulting with the research team, they decided to go out and collect data door to door. They would ask the residents questions and record their responses electronically. Four members of the team each took 25 addresses and set out to collect data.

At her first stop, Vanetta noticed several flowerpots with saucers underneath them full of stagnant water at the edge of the driveway. When she spoke with the resident, he said he tried to fill out the survey, but was confused. He and his wife rent this house and so it is not "their property." Yes, he had some of the items on the checklist, but he did not own the yard or the house. He thought he should forward the survey to his landlord, but he never got around to it. He also told Vanetta that most of the houses on the street were rentals. As she made her way down the street, the residents reported similar stories. Yes, they did have birdbaths and some discarded tires around, but it was not their property. They took the wording of the question literally. The other members of the research team got similar responses.

After collecting data from most of the residents in the neighborhood, Vanetta was confident that they had valid responses for analysis. From this project, she learned a valuable lesson as a researcher. First, she should have gotten to know the community a little better before implementing the survey. Simple demographics, such as home ownership, would have been helpful. Second, she did not pilot test her survey. She did not even think about how residents might perceive the wording of the checklist question if they were homeowners versus renters. In hindsight, she knew a small pilot test with neighborhood residents could have saved time and resources. In fact, engaging community residents along the entire process would have been beneficial. Before moving to the next phase of this project, she planned to meet with neighborhood stakeholders and hold an informational meeting with residents at the local library. Their input, as she learned, was vital to program success.

Critical Thinking Questions

1. How else could have the data on mosquito control have been collected?
2. What else should have been included during the planning phases of this project?
3. What other ways could you ask the question about the presence of standing water could collect?
4. What are some ways that Vanetta and her team could have included neighborhood residents in planning and implementing the survey?
5. In what ways does "citizen science" help public health research? What are some disadvantages of this data collection method?
6. What objective data might have been useful for this project?

COUNCIL ON EDUCATION FOR PUBLIC HEALTH FOUNDATIONAL KNOWLEDGE AND COMPETENCIES

Foundational Knowledge
Profession and Science of Public Health
- Explain the critical importance of evidence in advancing public health knowledge.

Foundational Competencies
Evidence-Based Approaches to Public Health
- Select quantitative and qualitative data-collection methods appropriate for a given public health context.

Planning and Management to Promote Health
- Assess population needs, assets, and capabilities that affect communities' health.
- Select methods to evaluate public health programs.

REFERENCES

1. Mosca I, Bhuachalla BN, Kenny RA. Explaining significant differences in subjective and objective measures of cardiovascular health: evidence for the socioeconomic gradient in a population-based study. *BMC Cardiovasc Disord.* 2013;13:64. doi:10.1186/1471-2261-13-64

2. Physical Activity Guidelines Advisory Committee. *2018 Physical Activity Guidelines Advisory Committee scientific report.* Washington, DC: U.S. Department of Health and Human Services; 2018. Accessed August 29, 2018. https://health.gov/sites/default/files/2019-09/PAG_Advisory_Committee_Report.pdf

3. Troiano R, Berrigan D, Dodd K, et al. Physical activity in the United States measured by accelerometer. *Med Sci Sports Exerc.* 2008;40(1):181–188. doi:10.1249/mss.0b013e31815a51b3

4. Bailey EJ, Malecki KC, Engelman CD, et al. Predictors of discordance between perceived and objective neighborhood data. *Ann Epidemiol.* 2014;24(3):214–221. doi:10.1016/j.annepidem.2013.12.007

5. Dillman DA, Smyth JD, Christian LM. *Internet, Phone, Mail, and Mixed-Mode Surveys: The Tailored Design Method.* Hoboken NJ: Wiley; 2014.

6. Centers for Disease Control and Prevention. Behavioral Risk Factor Surveillance System. Accessed September 23, 2019. https://www.cdc.gov/brfss/index.html

7. Blumberg SJ, Luke J V. Wireless substitution: early release of estimates from the national health interview survey, January–June 2018. 2018. Accessed August 6, 2019. https://www.cdc.gov/nchs/data/nhis/earlyrelease/wireless201812.pdf

8. Hiya Corporation. State of the call report: how we use our mobile phones in the era of robocalls. n.d. Accessed September 20, 2019. https://hiya.com/blog/2019/01/29/state-of-the-call-report-mobile-phones-in-the-era-of-robocalls

9. Gustat J, O'Malley K, Hu T, et al. Support for physical activity policies and perceptions of work and neighborhood environments: variance by BMI and activity status at the county and individual levels. *Am J Health Promot.* 2014;28(suppl 3):S33-S43. doi:10.4278/ajhp.130430-QUAN-216

10. U.S. Postal Service. A decade of facts and figures.Postal facts. Accessed August 6, 2019. https://facts.usps.com/table-facts

11. U.S. Office of the Inspector General. Millennials and the mail. Accessed September 20, 2019. https://www.uspsoig.gov/sites/default/files/document-library-files/2018/RARC-WP-18-011.pdf

12. Institute for Social Research. Health and retirement study. Accessed September 23, 2019. https://hrs.isr.umich.edu/about

13. Pew Research Center. 10% of Americans don't use the internet:who are they? Factank: news in the numbers. 2019. Accessed August 6, 2019. https://www.pewresearch.org/fact-tank/2019/04/22/some-americans-dont-use-the-internet-who-are-they

14. Centers for Medicare and Medicaid Services. Ambulatory Surgical Center (ACS) Infection Control Surveyor Worksheet. n.d. Accessed September 22, 2019. Retrieved from https://www.cms.gov/Regulations-and-Guidance/Guidance/Manuals/downloads/som107_exhibit_351.pdf

15. Mckenzie TL, Cohen DA. SOPARC (System for Observing Play and Recreation in Communities) description and procedures manual. January 10, 2006. Accessed August 6, 2019. https://activeliving research.org/sites/activelivingresearch.org/files/SOPARC_Protocols.pdf

16. McKenzie TL. SOPLAY system for observing play and leisure activity in youth description and procedures manual. January 10, 2006. Accessed August 6, 2019. https://activelivingresearch.org/sites/activelivingresearch.org/files/SOPLAY_Protocols.pdf

17. Mckenzie TL. SOFIT (System for Observing Fitness Instruction Time) description and procedures manual (Generic Version for Paper Entry). May 1, 2015. Accessed August 6, 2019. https://activeliving research.org/sites/activelivingresearch.org/files/SOFIT_Protocols_05.01.15.pdf

18. Nutrition Environment Measures Survey. The NEMS tools. 2018. Accessed August 6, 2019. https://www.med.upenn.edu/nems/measures.shtml

19. Pless R, Jacobs N. AMOS: project overview. 2015. Accessed August 6, 2019. http://amos.cse.wustl.edu

20. Hipp JA, Manteiga A, Burgess A, et al. Webcams, crowdsourcing, and enhanced crosswalks: developing a novel method to analyze active transportation. *Front Public Health*. 2016;4:97. doi:10.3389/fpubh.2016.00097

21. Wazny K. Applications of crowdsourcing in health: an overview. *J Glob Health*. 2018;8(1). doi:10.7189/JOGH.08.010502

22. Harris J, Mansour R, Choucair B, et al. Health department use of social media to identify foodborne Illness—Chicago, Illinois, 2013–2014. *MMWR*. 2014;63(32):681–685. Accessed September 23, 2019. https://www.cdc.gov/mmwr/preview/mmwrhtml/mm6332a1.htm

23. Quade P, Nsoesie EO. A platform for crowdsourced foodborne Illness surveillance: description of users and reports. *JMIR Public Health Surveill*. 2017;3(3):e42. Accessed September 23, 2019. doi:10.2196/publichealth.7076

24. Marlar J. Using text messaging to reach survey respondents. Gallup Methodology Blog. November 1, 2017. https://news.gallup.com/opinion/methodology/221159/using-text-messaging-reach-survey-respondents.aspx

25. U.S. Department of Health and Human Services, Office of Minority Health. The National CLAS Standards. 2019. Accessed September 6, 2020. https://minorityhealth.hhs.gov/omh/browse.aspx?lvl=2&lvlid=53

26. Moorhead A, Bond R, and Zheng H. Smart food: Crowdsourcing of experts in nutrition and non-experts in identifying calories of meals using smartphone as a potential tool contributing to obesity prevention and management. 2015 *IEEE International Conference on Bioinformatics and Biomedicine (BIBM)*. Washington, DC. November 9–12, 2015:1777–1779. doi:10.1109/BIBM.2015.7359959

ADDITIONAL READINGS AND RESOURCES

Jacobs N, Burgin W, Fridrich N, et al. The global network of outdoor webcams: properties and applications. GIS '09 Proceedings of the 17th ACM SIGSPATIAL International Conference on the Advances in Geographic Information Systems; 111–120, 2009. Accessed September 23, 2019. http://cs.uky.edu/~jacobs/papers/jacobs09gis.pdf

U.S. Census Bureau. Race: about. 2018. Accessed September 6, 2020. https://www.census.gov/topics/population/race/about.html

Quantitative Data Analysis

The way we work in public health is, we make the best recommendations and decisions based on the best available data.

—Tom Frieden, MD, CEO, Resolve to Save Lives

LEARNING OBJECTIVES

After reading this chapter, the reader will be able to

- Understand how to plan for quantitative data analysis.
- Choose appropriate statistical tests.
- Describe the results of statistical analysis.
- Describe statistical and practical significance of research results.

INTRODUCTION

Quantitative data analysis is the phase in the research process during which numbers are transformed into meaningful statistics. However, the analysis phase of the research process is not the first time a public health researcher should think about analyzing quantitative data. Analysis is informed by several phases prior to this one. The literature review provides insight into the pros and cons of analytic methods used for the topic of interest. Also, your data-collection tools, the characteristics of the data, and the size of your sample all influence how you analyze quantitative data. Your analysis may be univariate, bivariate, or multivariate (Exhibit 10.1), or a combination of these types.

EXHIBIT 10.1 TYPES OF QUANTITATIVE DATA ANALYSIS

UNIVARIATE	BIVARIATE	MULTIVARIATE
One variable	Two variables	Two or more variables
Descriptive	Determines relationship	Determines concurrent relationship
Examples:	Examples:	Examples:
Age	Gender and BMI	Smoking status by age and gender
Gender	Income and Health Status	Physical activity by zip code and BMI
Educations		

BMI, body mass index.

Once you have raw data, there are several key steps needed to prepare for analysis. The literature sometimes refers to this phase as *cleaning and editing* the data. Quantitative analysis is based on analyzing numbers or numeric codes. Qualitative data, discussed in Chapter 11, Qualitative Study Designs; Chapter 12, Qualitative Data Collection; and Chapter 13, Qualitative Data Analysis, is generally based on words, and analysis methodology is very different from data represented by numbers. Assigning numeric codes to data is the first step in editing raw data. For example, response options to a question on general health status might be coded as follows:

Question 1: Would you say your health in general is . . .

Response	Numeric Code
Excellent	1
Very Good	2
Good	3
Fair	4
Poor	5
Don't Know	999

In the previous question, "999" corresponds to "don't know." Be sure to use a numeric code for the "don't know" category that cannot be a valid response and use a consistent "don't know" numeric code across all variables. When the process of numeric coding is complete, information should be recorded into a **data codebook**. A codebook is a quantitative guide to your data. It documents the specific meaning assigned to each variable, and serves as a reference guide for the research team throughout analysis and interpretation. The codebook evolves through the analysis process. Each time a new variable is created, it should be added to the codebook. Many statistical software programs can also easily print a codebook of all variables in your current dataset. New variables can be developed by recoding a variable into different categories, or transformed by combining or calculating existing variable information. If you wanted to collapse some of the response categories in the general-health question example, you could recode into an additional variable as:

Question 1: Would you say your health in general is . . .

Response	Original Numeric Code	Recode
Excellent	1	1
Very Good	2	1
Good	3	1
Fair	4	2
Poor	5	2
Don't Know	999	999

Now the response categories are dichotomous (1 and 2), with only two levels for analysis (Good/Very Good/Excellent and Fair/Poor) instead of five. Age, for example, is often recoded into categories. Continuous variables, such as age, are commonly recoded into categories for analysis. Depending on your research question, it may be more helpful to know that almost 50% of your sample is under the age of 10 years than it is to know that the mean age is 11.5. Transforming individual variables into total scale scores is also common in research. For example, the responses to five individual questions on social support may be added together into a sum score of social support. Recoding or transforming the data should be guided by theory, past literature, or the methods needed to answer the research question.

Another necessary step in preparing the data for analysis is to identify any cases that do not fit within the intended population. Suppose you were interested in perceptions of healthy meals from mothers with children under the age of 5. You ask a qualifying question on the survey to ensure respondents meet the criteria of having at least one young child, but there are a few cases for which the respondent indicated no children. These cases should be omitted in analysis. Document the number of cases omitted and the reasons for their exclusion. Keeping track of actions during this preanalysis phase is helpful when writing the Methods section of a research report.

Addressing missing data is also important in preparing data for analysis. Respondents may intentionally or unintentionally skip questions. Look for patterns in variables with missing data. Perhaps the question was unclear or not meaningful to participants. (Pilot testing questions may help avoid this.) If the missing values are not managed properly, the researcher may end up with an inaccurate interpretation of the data. Common statistical techniques used to estimate the missing values include regression, maximum likelihood estimation, and multiple data imputation. Consult with a biostatistician on the best ways to handle missing variables specific to your data.

Many survey questions offer a "don't know" response option. These responses should not be considered missing data. The pattern of "don't know" responses may tell a unique story about the respondent group, and percentages of "don't know" should be reported along with other percentages of other choices.

HOW MUCH IS MISSING?

How complete must a case be in order to keep the data for analysis? Sometimes people skip questions or just do not finish the survey. Certainly, if the key questions are not answered, the case would not be useful for analysis. For instance, if the key component of your research question has to do with gender differences and a respondent does not indicate gender, that case should be omitted. Partial completion is another issue. If a respondent only answers seven of 10 survey questions, should that case be included? What if you need a certain number of cases for multivariate analysis? There is no standard answer. Look for patterns in characteristics of the missing data. Explore common ways to replace missing data if you choose to keep them in your data set. Be sure to document the rationale for managing partially completed cases.

DESCRIPTIVE STATISTICS

Descriptive statistics summarize the basic features or characteristics of the data, and these summaries are the basis of most quantitative analyses. Frequencies are descriptive statistics in the simplest form. Frequency summaries provide the numbers of cases within selected categories, and percentage of cases within the total sample. These summaries help to identify any outliers or out-of-range responses within the data. Table 10.1 shows a frequency table of characteristics of sample data. In quickly scanning the table, you can see three fourths (75%) of the sample were men, the Midwest region was least represented, over half were Republican, and most had between 1 and 10 years in the position. Frequency tables provide a quick snapshot of the data and are a necessary part of a research report.

Frequencies can also be used to describe the relationship between two variables. Cross-tabulations present the data summaries in a way that shows relationships between categories of the variables. An example of a cross-tabulation is presented in Table 10.2. This table shows

TABLE 10.1 EXAMPLE OF A FREQUENCY TABLE

Variable	n (%)
Gender of mayor	
Female	14 (24.6)
Male	43 (75.4)
Region	
Northeast	20 (35.1)
Midwest	7 (12.3)
South	15 (26.3)
West	15 (26.3)

(continued)

TABLE 10.1 EXAMPLE OF A FREQUENCY TABLE (*continued*)	
Variable	*n* (%)
Political party	
Democrat	21 (36.8)
Republican	31 (54.4)
Independent	05 (08.8)
Years in position	
Less than 1 year	8 (14.1)
1–5 years	22 (38.5)
6–10 years	20 (35.1)
More than 10 years	7 (12.3)
	57 = *N*

the breakdown of specialization and category of employment for a sample of 1,000 graduates of a public health program. The table shows the majority of the sample specialized in epidemiology and most of those were employed in health departments. The majority of those specializing in health policy were employed in government. Graduates specializing in health behavior were almost equally represented across the four employment categories.

Measures of central tendency is a category of descriptive statistics used to indicate how the data clusters around the "center" location of the distribution. The most common measures of central tendency are the mean, median, and mode. The **mean** is the sum of the values of observations divided by the number of evaluations. It is the most commonly reported measure of central tendency. The **median** is the middle value in the ranked distribution of values in a set of observations. Because outliers or extreme values within the data can affect the mean, the median is also important to report. The **mode** is the value that most often occurs in the set of observations. Table 10.3 shows a sample set of data with calculations of the mean, median, and mode.

Even though calculating the mean, median, and mode reduces data into three meaningful statistics, the data has more of a story to tell. Another category of descriptive statistics is **measures of dispersion. Dispersion** shows the distribution of values around the mean or some other central value. For example, **range** is a measure of dispersion outlining the difference between the lowest and the highest values within a variable. In most data, the greater the range, the higher the variability. *Variability* refers to how spread out or clustered data is around the central point. However, the presence of outliers can affect the interpretation of the range. From the data in Table 10.3, the range of number of children is 0 to 7. In this example, if one of the families had 10 children, the range would be inflated by this one case. **Standard deviation** is a commonly used measure of dispersion. A standard pattern is normal distribution (normal or bell curve) where the data are symmetrically dispersed, clustered around the mean and tapering off further away from the mean on each end of the curve. In a normal distribution, 68% of the data points fall between +1 and −1 standard deviations from the mean (Figure 10.1). About 95% are between +2 and −2 standard deviations from the mean, with 99%

TABLE 10.2 EXAMPLE OF A CROSS-TABULATION TABLE

Graduate Specialization of Public Health Program and Employment (N = 1,000)

	Epidemiology n = 456	Health Behavior n = 267	Health Policy (n = 154)	Environmental Health (n = 123)
Employment				
Health Dept.	172	68	21	32
Corporate	102	60	39	54
Government	117	63	70	10
Nonprofit	65	77	44	27
	456	267	154	123

TABLE 10.3 MEAN, MEDIAN, AND MODE FREQUENCIES OF NUMBER OF CHILDREN OF FAMILIES IN THE HEALTH INTERVENTION

Number of Children N = 585	Number of Families in Each Category N = 250
0	27
1	54
2	79
3	43
4	22
5	10
6	8
7	7

Note: Mean = 2.3, median = 2, mode = 2.

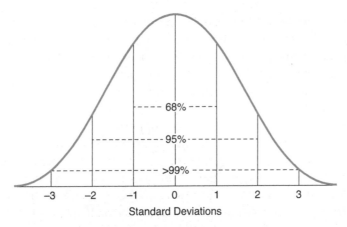

FIGURE 10.1 **Normal distribution curve.**

of the data between +3 and −3 standard deviations from the mean. Data can fall into non-normal distribution patterns. For example, the distribution can be skewed (asymmetrical), or bimodal with two peaks. **Interquartile range** is another measure of dispersion, which is the difference between the first and third quartiles, identifying the middle 50% of the data. Dispersion patterns help describe the data and inform statistical testing.

INFERENTIAL STATISTICS

Inferential statistics take descriptive statistics to another level. With **inferential statistics,** we can draw conclusions about a whole population based on results from a sample of that population. In other words, we identify the extent to which we can "infer" the findings from one study to the larger population. Inferential statistics are based on probability theory. Probability theory examines the pattern of results from repeating an event (e.g., coin toss) many times to determine whether the outcome is random or typical. Probability quantifies the uncertainty of events and how likely it is that results would have occurred in certain circumstances, and places results in a theoretical distribution pattern and distribution. Inferential statistics inform the interpretation of data, and quantifies the dependability of the findings in the context of the broader population.

Hypothesis Testing

In Chapter 4, Operationalization and Measurement, we presented hypothesis development. Not all research studies have hypotheses, but if the study aims to test a relationship among concepts, we can use quantitative data analysis to prove hypotheses are correct or incorrect. Many studies are guided by more than one hypothesis. Research studies may include an experimental or research hypothesis and an alternative hypothesis. The alternative hypothesis specifies the relationship that will emerge as true if the research hypothesis is proven not to be true. An alternative hypothesis may be a null hypothesis, referring to no difference between groups of study.

We use inferential statistics to test the hypotheses. The results of these tests are the determination of statistical significance, a measure of the likelihood that the results are due to chance. Inferential statistics are used to calculate *p* **values**, or the probability of obtaining the results by chance (ranges 0–1). The researcher compares the *p* value to a level of significance set prior to analysis. A common significance level in public health research is .05. This represents a one-in-20 chance that the observation is incorrect. A more stringent significance level (.01) can be used, where there is a one-in-100 chance that the observation is wrong. When the analysis results in a *p* value lower than the set significance level, there is more confidence the relationship is less likely due to chance. With this information the research hypothesis, alternative hypothesis, or the null hypothesis can be supported or rejected.

Inferential statistics improve confidence in interpretation of results, but probability means that no test is 100% certain. For example, two types of errors may occur (Table 10.4.). **Type I error** is the probability of rejecting the null hypothesis when it is in fact true. The chance for this error coincides with the statistical significance level. If it is set at .05, the probability of type I error is 5%. A stricter criterion (e.g., .01) reduces type 1 error. If you accept the null hypothesis as true, there is also a chance of error, called **type II error**. Type II error occurs when you retain the null hypothesis when it is false. Study design can address the risk of type II error. Designing a study with high power minimizes the risk of type II error. **Power** refers to the ability to correctly detect statistical significance, or reject the null hypothesis when it is false. Using larger sample sizes and measuring stronger effect size increases power, thus reducing the chance of type II error. Power calculations (presented in Chapter 5, Sampling) justify and quantify the most appropriate sample size for the measurement of effect relevant to the concept of interest.

Researching complex public health topics requires looking at the issues and studying the results in more than one way. Statistical significance is just one part of quantitative data analysis. There are also measures of **effect size**, or the strength of the effect of a variable on the outcome. For example, how much variability in a person's willingness to get a flu shot (dependent variable) is due to a vaccination campaign (independent variable)? The effect size is reported as a percentage, and if the effect size for the flu shot example is .15, then 15% of the variability in a person's willingness to get a flu shot is accounted for by the intervention. Study results can show statistical significance, but low effect sizes, especially in extremely large samples. Although it is unlikely that an independent variable will explain all of the variability in a dependent variable, the larger the effect size, the stronger the evidence to support the relationship.

Confidence intervals describe the margin of error. The confidence interval represents a range with an upper and lower number calculated from sample data. Confidence intervals will contain the outcome measure (e.g., population mean) a specified proportion of the time. Typically, the interval is computed at 95%, meaning 95% of the time, the confidence interval contains the outcome. Confidence intervals do not reflect the probability of containing the outcome. The wider the range of the confidence interval, the less precise the interpretation.

TABLE 10.4 TYPE I AND TYPE II ERRORS IN HYPOTHESIS TESTING

Type I Error	Type II Error
Reject H_0 when it is true	Fail to reject H_0 when it is false
Incorrectly determine that a relationship exists	Incorrectly determine that there is **no** relationship when one really exists
False positive	False negative

PARAMETRIC AND NONPARAMETRIC TESTS

There are many different statistical tests used in quantitative data analysis, and data characteristics determine which test is most appropriate. The measurement level of the variables is one example. Some tests are applicable for nominal data, but limited by the number of categories within the variable. Other tests can only be used with interval or ratio data. These limitations make it important to plan for analysis when developing data-collection strategies. In some instances, data can be recoded to fit the requirements of a test. For example, the continuous, ratio data from the question "How much did you spend on weight-loss products this week?" could be recoded into categories such as: 0$, 1$ to 20$, 21$ to 30$, 31$+. Another characteristic of the data affecting test selection is distribution. This makes descriptive statistics an important first step in testing for statistical significance. In addition, there are distinct procedural differences based on the number of variables in the analysis. Bivariate (two variables) or multivariate (more than two variables) analyses require different tests.

Two broad categories of statistical significance tests are parametric and nonparametric tests. Explanations of these two categories can fill textbooks, but only a brief summary is presented in this section. Simply stated, the main factor in choosing between using parametric or nonparametric tests is based on whether the mean or median is a better measure of central tendency in your data. Parametric tests are used when assumptions are made about the "parameters," or properties and distribution of the sample population. Parametric tests are used when the mean is a better descriptor of the data distribution than the median. Parametric tests are used when the dependent variable is interval or ratio data. Nonparametric tests are not dependent on assumptions about the parameters or distribution of the data, but instead make assumptions about sampling and the independence or dependence of the samples. Nonparametric tests rely on the median (rather than the mean) of the data.

There are three main assumptions for parametric testing. The first assumption is that the concept or characteristic of interest is normally distributed within the study population. Second, there is a homogeneity of variance, meaning the amount of difference among the population varies equally between groups. Third, parametric tests assume each observation being compared is independent of any other observation. There are statistical procedures for testing these assumptions to guide analyses. If the data do not meet the assumptions for parametric testing, using parametric procedures will likely result in inaccurate results. Good experimental design with careful consideration to analysis type is necessary to determine the appropriate test choice.

Three common parametric tests are the independent samples t test, analysis of variance (ANOVA), and Pearson's correlation. Table 10.5 outlines a summary of these tests. An independent samples **t test** compares the means of the dependent variable for an independent variable with two independent groups. This test will indicate statistical significance, based on the difference in means. You should select this test only when the mean of your data best represents the variables distribution. The independent variable can be nominal or ordinal with only two levels, and the dependent variable needs to be an interval or ratio. **ANOVA** is a parametric test statistic similar to a t test, in which the means of an interval or ratio dependent variable are compared with an independent variable, but the independent variable can be dichotomous or have multiple categories. The result of ANOVA is an F-statistic. As with a t test, ANOVA shows statistical significance based on mean differences among groups.

TABLE 10.5 SUMMARY OF COMMONLY USED PARAMETRIC AND NONPARAMETRIC TESTS				
Statistical Test	Independent Variable	Dependent Variable	Example Study Question	Notes
t test (t)	Nominal or ordinal with only two levels or attributes	Interval or ratio	Is there a significant difference between boys and girls on a measure of stress?	Compares the means (of the DV) for an IV of two groups Indicates statistical significance but not strength of relationship
ANOVA (F)	Nominal or ordinal with greater than or equal to two levels or attributes	Interval or ratio	Is there a significant difference in nutrition knowledge among students in three different classes?	Compares the means (of the DV) for an IV of two or more groups Indicates statistical significance but not strength of relationship
Pearson's correlation (r)	Interval or ratio	Interval or ratio	Is there a significant relationship between years since MPH degree and score of technology competence?	Assesses both statistical significance and the strength of association between two variables
Chi-square (χ²)	Nominal or ordinal with greater than or equal to two levels or attributes	Nominal or ordinal with greater than or equal to two levels or attributes	Is there a significant relationship between gender and smoking status?	Assesses whether the observed distributions differ significantly from the expected distributions Indicates statistical significance but not strength of relationship

ANOVA, analysis of variance; DV, dependent variable; IV, independent variable.

Pearson's correlation test assesses both statistical significance and strength of association/ relationship between two interval- or ratio-level variables. Pearson's r statistic can have a range from +1 to −1, where 0 means no association between the two variables. A negative value implies a negative correlation and a positive value shows a positive correlation. If the r value is closer to +1 or −1, the stronger the positive or negative association.

When parametric assumptions are not met, we can use non-parametric tests. Most non-parametric tests do not limit variables to interval or ratio levels of measurement. These tests can be applied to nominal or ordinal data that are not normally distributed. One example of a commonly used nonparametric test in public health research is the **chi-square test.** Chi-square (χ^2) assesses whether the observed distributions differ significantly from the expected distributions. Other nonparametric options for nonnormal data distribution include Mann–Whitney U Test (instead of independent samples t test, Kruskal–Wallis H test (instead of ANOVA), and Spearman correlation (instead of Pearson's correlation).

Good research design with careful consideration to analysis type is necessary to determine the appropriate test choice. Because data can be complicated, it is best to get expert advice if you are unsure about your analysis plan. It is much easier to address potential analysis issues earlier in the research process than later.

OTHER NOTES ON QUANTITATIVE ANALYSIS

There are issues other than test choice to consider in quantitative data analysis. How will your results add to the greater body of evidence on the topic? As indicated in Chapter 3, Ethics in Public Health Research, there are many population groups underrepresented in research. Even though researchers may be inclusive in their study samples, they often neglect to analyze data in a way that separates the groups. In order to promote health equity, we need to know whether interventions are equally effective across characteristics such as race/ethnicity, gender, or education. Plan your analysis to best reflect diversity.

Another issue related to quantitative data analysis is ethical interpretation and representation of findings. For this you need a comprehensive understanding of what the statistical results mean, and must correctly translate numbers into accurate reports. Do not overstate results, and include truthful limitations of the study. If all of your analyses result in nonsignificant findings, that is what needs to be reported. Choosing only to report favorable outcomes is unethical and may misrepresent analysis. Omitting nonsignificant or unexpected outcomes also creates an inaccurate evidence base. Remember, the results of many studies are compiled to determine intervention or program effectiveness. Null findings add to the aggregate evidence and are important for developing recommendations and public health priorities.

In addition to statistical significance, it is essential to report practical significance. Statistical significance does not reflect the importance of the results of the research evidence. **Practical significance** is an interpretation of whether the statistical significance is valuable in a practical sense. It helps answer the question: *Are these results useful in real life?* Although effect sizes can tell us the magnitude of difference and t tests show the relationship between variables, interpretation must go beyond statistical significance. More about translation and dissemination of results is available in Chapter 14, Summarizing and Visualizing Data, and in Chapter 15, Disseminating Research Results.

CHAPTER DISCUSSION QUESTIONS

1. Discuss the pros and cons of measuring and analyzing age as a continuous variable and a categorical variable. What factors should you consider in your measurement choice?
2. Why are descriptive statistics of key importance in quantitative data analysis?
3. How can data analysis be incorporated into all phases of the research process?
4. Discuss the potential ramification of researchers neglecting to analyze results of a study on effectiveness of a diabetes-prevention program by racial/ethnic group?
5. Describe the difference between statistical and practical significance.

RESEARCH PROJECT CHECK-IN

What to Do with All the Data

Completing data collection can feel like a relief, but there is still a lot of work yet to do. If you used paper surveys, you will need to enter the data into a database. For online surveys, the data will need to be transferred into the statistical analysis software program of your choosing. Go through the data and look for out-of-range responses or missing data. Use best practices for data management and be sure to keep track of all your data editing. You may be asked to justify what you did, and recording it reduces the burden on your memory. Your research question or study aim, along with the type of measurement used, should guide the type of analysis you will do. Be sure to accurately analyze, record, and interpret the statistical tests.

PUBLIC HEALTH RESEARCH METHODS IN REAL LIFE

It Is a Matter of Categorization

Maura was hired to provide epidemiological and biostatistical expertise on projects contracted through a small consultant firm. She was given data from a national health survey and asked to parse out some important information on correlates of women's physical and mental health related to motherhood. She was advised to recode the main continuous variables into categories for logistic regression analysis. The dependent variable was "number of days in the past month feeling unwell." The respondents to the survey recorded a number from 0 to 30. Because the client wanted logistic regression, Maura had to decide how to dichotomize this information. She ran descriptive statistics on the 1,000 responses and found the mean number of unwell days reported was 4, with a range of 0 to 15. She wondered how this compared with other national survey data. She found some information online that reported the average number of unwell days for the general population (both men and women) as 3.6. Because these results were similar to her data set, Maura decided the dependent variable would be comprised of two levels: less than the average number of unwell days (0–3) and above the average of unwell days (4+).

The next challenge was to figure out how to capture chronic conditions for this analysis. The survey asked a series of questions about eight main chronic conditions such as heart disease, diabetes, cancer, and arthritis. There were also two questions assessing the diagnosis of depression and anxiety. Given the overall aims of the study, Maura determined that mental and physical health should be assessed separately, then potentially combined or analyzed using the interaction between these two variables. She looked to the literature for ideas on how to recode these chronic conditions as each question about the conditions had a yes/no answer. She created a new variable for physical health conditions, which was a total number of "yes" responses to the eight physical health conditions questions. When she ran descriptive statistics, the mean was 2, with a range of 0 to 5. She used this information along with what she found in the literature and developed a new variable with categories of 0, 1, 2, 3+. Now she had to figure out how to recode the mental health conditions data. She created a cumulative variable for the depression-and-anxiety question responses. The new variable had a range of 0 to 2, with no anxiety or depression reported, either anxiety or depression reported, or both anxiety and depression reported. This would be the variable she would use in analysis.

As a final step, Maura had to figure out how to categorize the number of children reported in the data. The survey asked women to respond with the number and ages of the children living at home. She knew from experience that being a mother to children of any age is challenging, but she was not sure how to create a number/age variable for a meaningful analysis. She looked into other studies on women with children and found several relevant articles. One of the articles had a link to an online copy of the survey and data-management methods. She also read several systematic reviews on women's health related to motherhood. From this research, Maura decided to try it two ways. First, she just used number of children under the age of 18 living at home to develop a new categorical variable. The mean number of children reported in this dataset was 2, with a range of 0 to 7. The categories she created were 0, 1, 2, 3+. Next she created a variable on number of children under the age of 5 living at home. Her justification for this variable was many children go to kindergarten at age 5, so at 0 to 4, they would need a different level of care. She also decided to create another variable for number of children between the ages of 0 to 3 years. This category was commonly used in the literature, with categories of 0, 1, 2, 3+.

She could now begin the analysis and provide insight into the topic of correlates of mental and physical health among mothers. She knows data analysis is an iterative process and that she will likely have to recode and create even more variables, but this is a good start.

Critical Thinking Questions

1. Using descriptive data and past literature are two ways to inform the way in which variables are recoded. What other factors or resources should be considered?
2. Do you agree with the way Maura dichotomized the dependent variable in this example? Why or why not? If not, propose a different strategy.
3. How might categorizing continuous data hinder comparison of results across studies? What does this do to the cumulation of evidence?
4. What other ways could Maura have categorized the number and age of children?
5. What limitations may result from the way the variables in this example were categorized? What strategies could have been applied to reduce the limitations?

COUNCIL ON EDUCATION FOR PUBLIC HEALTH FOUNDATIONAL KNOWLEDGE AND COMPETENCIES

Foundational Knowledge

Profession and Science of Public Health

- Explain the critical importance of evidence in advancing public health knowledge.
- Explain the role of quantitative and qualitative methods and sciences in describing and assessing a population's health.

Foundational Competencies

Evidence-Based Approaches to Public Health

- Select quantitative and qualitative data collection methods appropriate for a given public health context.
- Analyze quantitative and qualitative data using biostatistics, informatics, computer-based programming, and software, as appropriate.
- Interpret results of data analysis for public health research, policy, or practice.

ADDITIONAL READINGS AND RESOURCES

Altman DG, Royston P. The cost of dichotomizing continuous variables. *BMJ*. 2006;332:1080. doi:10.1136/bmj.332.7549.1080

Gallo A. A refresher on statistical significance. *Harv Bus Rev*. February 16, 2016. Accessed October 2, 2019. https://hbr.org/2016/02/a-refresher-on-statistical-significance

Kahn Academy. Statistical significance of experiment. 2020. Accessed October 5, 2019. https://www.khanacademy.org/math/ap-statistics/probability-ap/randomness-probability-simulation/v/statistical-significance-experiment.

Kraemer HC, Kupfer DJ. Size of treatment effects and their importance to clinical research and practice. *Biol Psychiatry*. 2005;59(11):990–996. doi:10.1016/j.biopsych.2005.09.014

McCartney K, Rosenthal R. Effect size, practical importance, and social policy for children. *Child Dev*. 2003;71:173–180. doi:10.1111/1467-8624.00131

IV

QUALITATIVE RESEARCH

This section is dedicated to qualitative research and outlines the importance of this method in public health research. Paralleling information presented in the previous section on quantitative methods, this section describes the basics of study designs, data collection, and data analysis. Chapter 11, Qualitative Study Designs, explains the different approaches to conducting qualitative research and compares and contrasts this method with quantitative methods. It also outlines quality and ethical issues in qualitative research. Chapter 12, Qualitative Data Collection, outlines common ways to collect qualitative data, such as individual and group interviews, content gathering, and observation. Chapter 13, Qualitative Data Analysis, provides guidance for conducting qualitative data analysis and presents options and strategies commonly used in public health research.

Qualitative Study Designs

*Not everything that can be counted counts, and not everything
that counts can be counted.*

—Albert Einstein

LEARNING OBJECTIVES

The reader will be able to

- Understand reasons for conducting qualitative research.
- Explain the basic approaches to qualitative research.
- Compare and contrast qualitative and quantitative research.
- Understand appropriate samples for qualitative studies.
- Describe ethical issues relevant to qualitative research.

INTRODUCTION

Qualitative research is a broad term encompassing many different approaches and methods. Simply described, **qualitative research** provides an in-depth understanding of a phenomenon in a natural setting. Rooted in the participant perspective, qualitative inquiry helps to understand behaviors, beliefs, experiences, or attitudes of individuals or groups.

Qualitative research originated in the discipline of anthropology over a century ago,[1] and has evolved into an important way to study public health issues. Early anthropological studies provided insight into culture, human development, and many other complex social phenomena. In the past, the scientific community often criticized early studies for lacking rigor, and relying on unsystematic and journalistic techniques. Over time, the field of qualitative research advanced into a more methodological, scientific approach. It is now accepted as an effective way to gather information and evidence across many disciplines. For instance, qualitative methods are commonly used in market research to guide development of new products, test advertising strategies, and gain an understanding of consumer motivation.[2] Architects also use qualitative methods to study perceptions of buildings and assess occupancy behaviors. In public health, qualitative research is used to describe perceptions of disease risk and barriers to healthy behaviors, as well as many other complex health topics. See Table 11.1 for examples of theoretical constructs that can be studied using qualitative methods. Table 11.2 shows examples of published public health studies in a wide range of topics that used qualitative methods.

The value of qualitative research to public health has increased over the past few decades. There is now guidance on using evidence from qualitative research in systematic reviews.[9] There is also an increased focus on qualitative research in public health practice, as qualitative research skills are a necessary tool for practitioners. Since 2016, the Council on Education for Public Health (CEPH) requires accredited schools and programs to train public health students to be competent in qualitative data collection methods and analysis.

APPROACHES TO QUALITATIVE RESEARCH

Approaches to qualitative research are complex, and information on each approach can fill its own textbook. This overview provides a summary of the main approaches that serve as the basis of understanding qualitative research. **Phenomenology** is a term describing a main philosophical paradigm or approach to qualitative research. The phenomenological approach emphasizes description or interpretation of subjective lived experiences and perspectives. Studies that have a phenomenological basis are useful for formative or pilot research in which subjective experiences can help shape more effective intervention components. Research questions that involve this approach would consider the essential meaning

TABLE 11.1 QUALITATIVE APPLICATIONS TO PUBLIC HEALTH	
Research question: What are the experiences of women with genetic markers for increased risk of breast cancer?	
Knowledge	What do they know about risk?
Meaning	How does knowledge impact their lives and experiences?
Social and cultural norms	How do they perceive their risk compared to others?
Social processes	How does their experience impact interaction and communication with family and friends?
Global view	How does their experience influence recommendations for policy or systems change?

TABLE 11.2 EXAMPLES OF QUALITATIVE PUBLIC HEALTH STUDIES

Topic	Citation	Brief Summary
Nutrition	DiSantis et al.[3]	DiSantis and colleagues used data from interviews and focus groups with a socioeconomically diverse sample of Black adults in four cities to obtain an understanding of food marketing variables.
Obesity	He et al.[4]	He and colleagues conducted in-depth interviews with Latinx church leaders to gain perspectives on childhood obesity and insights on obesity-prevention programming in faith-based community settings.
Smoking	Kegler et al.[5]	Kegler and colleagues conducted focus groups to understand perspectives, including barriers and facilitators, on smoke-free homes in five American Indian/Alaska Native communities.
HPV	Sledge et al.[6]	Sledge and colleagues used data from focus groups with men from three community colleges to learn how to effectively increase awareness and knowledge about HPV.
Physical activity	Gilbert et al.[7]	Gilbert and colleagues interviewed adults living in six rural communities to explore perceptions of physical activity and walking-trail use.
Vaccines	Nowak et al.[8]	Nowak and colleagues analyzed the development and content of flu vaccine communications for respondents'knowledge, attitudes, and beliefs.

HPV, human papillomavirus.

of some phenomenon. For example, a qualitative study about spousal caregiving might attempt to answer the question, "What is the essence of being a caregiver to a spouse with a chronic disease?"

A second approach used in qualitative research is **ethnography**. Similar to phenomenology, ethnography is a way for a researcher to understand a phenomenon through the eyes of the participants. Ethnographical data collection takes place in natural settings. The data are used to accurately and thoroughly describe the way in which a culture or group of people live and interpret the meaning of concepts. Ethnography is well suited for public health research. It can elucidate cultural influences on health behavior and frame relevant health issues holistically, considering their historical, economic, and political contexts.[10]

Examples of public health ethnographical topics include HIV, gun violence, worker safety, immigrant health, and others. Ethnographical methods could be used to answer a research question such as: "How do new teen mothers experience life transition in the context of returning to school?"

Grounded theory is another qualitative approach used in public health research. It is a method used to develop theory that is "grounded in data systematically gathered and analyzed."[11] One of the hallmarks of this method is constant comparative analysis. This means the researcher goes back and forth between data collection and analysis. As data are analyzed, themes and patterns develop. New cases or observations can add to or change the way these themes develop. Once the researcher perceives no additional insights from new observations, this process stops and analysis can be completed. This simplistic description does not do justice to the complexity of grounded theory qualitative research. Look to the resources listed at the end of the chapter to learn more about it. Grounded theory is applicable to qualitative public health studies. A public health study using grounded theory might be guided by the research question: "What factors impact policy makers' preferences for receiving information on public health topics?" In this example, the researcher might vary the sampling of policy makers to ensure a broad scope of insights. More about constant comparative analysis is presented in Chapter 13, Qualitative Data Analysis.

Case studies can be an effective way to gain information on a complex public health topic. This qualitative approach is an empirical, in-depth exploration of an individual or groups (i.e., cases) to make conclusions within a particular context.[12] Different disciplines vary in the way they frame case studies, and there is a lack of consensus about the distinctions of this approach. Case studies can be framed within an individual perspective, exploring concepts such as development, personality, and learning of one person. Public health studies are more likely to frame case study research within organizations or communities, or with a social perspective. See Table 11.3 for applications of case study approaches. Use of multiple case studies is also common in public health. This approach offers an effective way to compare and contrast concepts across communities, organizations, groups, or individuals. More about designing case studies is presented in Chapter 12, Qualitative Data Collection.

TABLE 11.3 EXAMPLES OF DIFFERENT CASE-STUDY APPROACHES IN PUBLIC HEALTH RESEARCH

Case-Study Approach	Research Question Example
Community	What is the impact of the implementation of a new clean indoor air policy?
Organization	How does indoor space influence employee health?
Group	What is the impact of new competencies for public health practice on new MPH graduates?
Event	How did a hurricane affect healthcare access?

MPH, Masters of public health.

Interventions intended to increase active travel to school are an evidence-based strategy to increase walking among students and reduce risks for traffic-related injury.[13] Active travel to school is a complex concept. Policies, infrastructure, behaviors, and culture can influence whether or not children walk or bike to school. Eyler et al. used a case-study approach to explore walk-to-school policies in elementary schools. They used data from interviews with parents, teachers, school officials, city planners, and public safety officials to make conclusions about these policies.[14] Although most groups supported active travel to school, reasons differed. For example, school officials wanted less parking lot congestion, but teachers mentioned better student focus after an active commute. Multiple sources of information can provide a more comprehensive conclusion than using a single source. Findings from case studies, such as this one. can be used to tailor interventions to match the various perspectives and priorities.

QUALITATIVE VERSUS QUANTITATIVE RESEARCH

Qualitative and quantitative research methods differ in several ways, beginning with the research purpose (Table 11.4). Qualitative methods are used in exploratory or descriptive research, whereas quantitative methods explain or evaluate issues. Qualitative studies often aim to describe, understand, explain, develop, or generate information on a topic. The rigid and systematic structure of quantitative methods allows researchers to quantify concepts and variations, or predict causal relationships. Quantitative research questions often include words such as *what?* and *how much?* instead of more qualitative inquiries such as *why?* and *how?* Epidemiologists use quantitative methods to determine how much disease or disease risk exists within a population. A public health researcher might use qualitative methods to find out more about the way in which people perceive the disease or its risk factors. Second, rather than testing and confirming hypotheses, qualitative research creates them. Conclusions from qualitative research provide meaning and context, which can be used to develop new ways of thinking about relationships, experiences, or norms within public health topics. Data collection differs between these two methods, too. Quantitative approaches rely on structured methods such as surveys or systematic, measured observations. Objective or closed-ended questions are commonly used. Qualitative research involves open-ended questions delivered through more personal interactions between researcher and the participant. Interviews, focus groups, or immersive observations result in rich and detailed data. Qualitative research allows participants to provide data in their own words, rather than forcing a fixed response. Consider the following question from the 2019 Youth Risk Behavior Survey (YRBS) on sleep:

On an average school night, how many hours of sleep do you get?
A. 4 or less hours
B. 5 hours
C. 6 hours
D. 7 hours
E. 8 hours
F. 9 hours
G. 10 or more hours

TABLE 11.4 COMPARISON OF QUALITATIVE AND QUANTITATIVE METHODS	
QUALITATIVE	**QUANTITATIVE**
Understanding	Explanation
Hypothesis or theory generating	Hypothesis or theory testing
Inductive	Deductive
Uses observation	Uses objectivity
How? Why? In what context?	What? How much?

This question asks participants to select a response from a list of choices. Analysis would likely include frequencies and percentages of each response. Qualitative methods might be used if you were more interested in what an average school night entails, such as the inquiry: *Describe what you do most weeknights during the school year.*

This elicits information on what might influence sleep patterns, not just the number of hours students sleep. Knowing how high school students spend their evening time would be helpful in developing curricula on sleep health.

As the sleep example suggests, data derived from quantitative (numbers) and qualitative methods (words) are very different, resulting in distinct analytic methodologies. The responses from the interview question could be transcribed and the resulting text is the data to be analyzed. The data derived from the YRBS question would have numerical values assigned to each response, and the values could be manipulated and analyzed to identify any statistical significance. There are no p values in qualitative research, but patterns and themes emerge instead.

ISSUES TO CONSIDER IN QUALITATIVE RESEARCH DESIGN

A good research design involves careful planning and adherence to research best practices. Scientific rigor in qualitative studies is characterized by the strength of the research design and the way in which the design and methods achieve the overall research goals. Qualitative studies should be designed to systematically and thoroughly gather, analyze, and interpret data so findings contribute to the current evidence of the study topic.

One major consideration when planning a qualitative research study is the sample population. Sampling in qualitative studies is not based on random selection of participants. The sample group should provide information that will contribute to the overall reserach goals. Similar to quantitative studies, samples in qualitative research can be based on certain characteristics (criterion sample). If your study topic is breastfeeding and working mothers, you will likely select employed (or previously employed) women with infants to provide you with your qualitative data. Targeted sampling is also commonly used in qualitative studies. You want to select a sample with enough knowledge about the topic to provide you with enough relevant data. If a qualitative study aimed to explore perception of care in a certain health center, the sample would be targeted within that health center. Snowball sampling, or participant-generated sampling, is a good method to use when the researcher is not familiar with the entire reach of a certain research topic. To explore the impact of a policy change on a community, researchers could start with a list of key informants, and then ask these informants for the names of other people who might be able to provide insight into the issue. If a qualitative study aims to compare and contrast concepts, researchers would include variants or deviant cases in the sample. A study on barriers to exercise might include regular exercisers and people who are sedentary.

Many qualitative approaches involve personal contact between participant and researcher, making access to the sample population a key design issue. Are there lists of organizations or people that can be used as the basis of qualitative sampling? Can you network or attend community meetings or get to know the population in ways so as to learn about whom might best fit your sampling needs? When planning a qualitative study, to facilitate access, it is necessary to build in time to learn about the population of interest.

How large of a sample do you need for qualitative research? The only consensus about sample size in the field of qualitative research is that it depends on the method being used and the unique characteristics of the study. The concept of **saturation** can inform sample size. When data reveals no new insights, or unique findings emerge, saturation is reached. A benefit to qualitative research is the flexibility between data collection and analysis. If the researcher feels as if they need to continue to collect data in order reach a point of saturation, additional sample numbers can be added, even after initial analysis. More on sample size recommendations for different types of qualitative data collection is presented in Chapter 12, Qualitative Data Collection.

One's timeline is also an important factor within qualitative research design. Researchers need to carefully build time for learning about the population and setting of interest early in the research process. This step can help in planning the timing of data collection. Proactively learning about any events or happenings that might affect data collection will be of tremendous benefit to the efficiency of the study. For example, it would not be a good idea to plan to conduct interviews with teachers during breaks for school holidays. Study designs should also provide adequate time for data collection and analysis (and potentially more data collection and analysis). Look to past studies or experienced qualitative researchers for advice on how to best plan a timeline.

Another issue important to qualitative research study design is **reflexivity**. Reflexivity refers to exploring (i.e., reflecting) how the perspectives of the researcher and the interaction between researcher and participant influence the research process. Because a researcher's background, characteristics, or experiences can affect processes and outcomes, a reflexive study design must include a plan for recording and reporting interactive factors throughout the study.

QUALITY IN QUALITATIVE RESEARCH STUDIES

Assessing the quality of most quantitative studies is straightforward, with use of well-accepted measures and parameters. The nature of qualitative studies warrants different criteria for evaluating quality. Reliability and validity measures of quantitative studies are not applicable to qualitative research, yet these concepts remain important to assess—albeit in different ways. Guba and Lincoln (1994) proposed alternative criteria for evaluating qualitative research. Characteristics of trustworthiness parallel reliability and validity in quantitative studies.[15] Trustworthiness involves establishing four factors:

1. **Credibility.** Parallel to internal validity, credibility refers to adhering to best practices for research. A credible study also includes respondent validation or member checking. The researcher should present findings back to those who were studied to ensure the truth of the interpretation.
2. **Transferability.** Transferability is similar to external validity. Qualitative studies are contextually unique, making it difficult to generalize findings to other populations or settings. However, it is the responsibility of the researcher to provide enough details so findings can be used to build evidence and inform other studies.
3. **Dependability.** Dependability is a way to promote reliability in qualitative studies. Carefully recording each step in the research process improves transparency and dependability. This also helps to justify inferences and conclusions from the data. Dependable studies show findings that are consistent and could be replicated. Analyzing qualitative data in a reliable way (e.g., using more than one person in data coding) is discussed further in Chapter 13, Qualitative Data Analysis.
4. **Confirmability.** Complete objectivity is not realistic in qualitative research. However, studies should be designed in a neutral way, so that findings are shaped by participants not the investigator's internal biases. Reflexivity is one way to improve confirmability of a qualitative study.

Triangulation, or using multiple data sources, can improve the trustworthiness of a qualitative study. Using more than one source of data can facilitate deeper understanding of a concept, and to check the consistency of findings against other data-collection methods. By using different data sources within the same method (e.g., collecting data in the same way, but at different time points or settings), triangulation can also add to the quality of a study. Another way to enhance trustworthiness is to use a team of researchers. Different people may contribute different views of observation and interpretation, reducing the impact of subjectivity and bias of a solo researcher.

ETHICS IN QUALITATIVE RESEARCH

There are ethical issues unique to qualitative research, which must be considered throughout the research process. Qualitative studies often involve greater connection between researcher and participants than quantitative studies, making the research process itself prone to ethical concerns. In addition, some risks to participants in qualitative studies may not be anticipated because methods can evolve over the course of the study. Researchers need to think carefully about safeguarding the participants in all study phases. The institutional review board process helps to document how ethical concerns will be addressed, but it is up to the research team to safeguard participants throughout the study.

Several steps in the research process create specific ethical vulnerabilities for participants. The following text outlines some potential concerns and suggestions for addressing them with best practices for ethical qualitative research.

Sampling and Recruitment

Qualitative methodologies are often used to reach very specific populations who may not be well represented in larger, quantitative studies. This specificity creates unique ethical challenges for sampling and recruitment. Researchers need to be knowledgeable about culture, characteristics, and vulnerabilities of their target population before the study begins. It is vital to learn about the history and reputation of research within the population or community of interest. As discussed in Chapter 3, Ethics in Public Health Research, unethical historical events may contribute to current mistrust about research. Building relationships before recruitment is vital to creating an environment of mutual respect and trust. Initial information presented in recruitment must include full disclosure of the research goals and expected outcomes. Researchers should outline how these outcomes can benefit those involved to help establish a trustworthy relationship.

Some qualitative studies are conducted within narrow contexts such as communities, organizations, or schools. People in these settings can be very connected to one another, increasing the risk of loss of confidentiality. This is especially a concern for research on sensitive topics. For example, snowball sampling may not be the best method to use when recruiting participants in cases where people might not want to be identified by the characteristic of study (e.g., HIV status). Allowing privacy for making the choice about study participation should also be provided in some cases.

As part of recruitment, researchers may want to collect personal information from participants such as address or other contact information. If monetary incentives are used, some institutional review boards require documentation of Social Security numbers. This may be of concern to vulnerable populations who may not wish to disclose this information for confidentiality reasons. Researchers need to know the potential for these issues prior to recruitment.

Mistrust about research can be present in many populations. To recruit women living in rural Missouri for a qualitative study about barriers to physical activity, Eyler et al. put advertisements in local newspapers and flyers about the study in places around town.[17] After 3 weeks, no one inquired about the study. The research team visited the community and spoke with key informants about the failed recruitment efforts. It seemed as if there was a mistrust of both the city (St. Louis) and university research in many rural communities. The fact that the recruitment ads were emblazoned with information about "outsiders" coming in to investigate this small community was an immediate cause for women to refuse participation. More effort was put into building relationships with people in the community in order to gain their trust, and eventually enough women were recruited for the focus groups. As this example shows, taking time to know the community and how its members perceive research is vital to a successful study.

Informed Consent and Data Collection

Ethical research includes getting informed consent of all participants. Informed consent must include the study details, what participation entails, risks, benefits, and anticipated outcomes. This information needs to be presented in a format relevant and comprehensible to the participant population. In qualitative studies, consent does not end with a signature on a form. It is an ongoing process throughout the study.

Data collection should be convenient to participants. Burden or inconvenience should be minimized. Past literature or gaining insight from researchers experienced with the population of interest can be valuable in informing this aspect of the study. Researchers should consider setting and privacy, but also other ways to reduce participant burden such as providing transportation or childcare during data collection.

Although it may be easy to understand voluntary participation and the having the choice to quit at any time when filling out an online survey, the personal interaction required of many qualitative methods (such as interviews) may necessitate more explicit consent. The researcher needs to convey trust and respect with participants, so if they do experience discomfort during data collection, they will be empowered to speak up or remove themselves from the study.

Unlike many quantitative data-collection techniques, anonymity in qualitative research is often difficult, so safeguards of confidentiality are of utmost importance. The participants need to know how they would be identified in analysis and research reports. Data collection via interviews and focus groups is often recorded by the researchers to aid in analysis. Some participants may not agree to this, so researchers must have other options available. For example, state legislators were not receptive to having interview conversations recorded in a study of childhood obesity policy. Two members of the research team took verbatim notes as an alternative to digital transcription from an audio recording.[16] It is an ethical necessity for the researcher to be sensitive to and address confidentiality concerns.

Interpretation and Reporting

A hallmark of qualitative data analysis is interpretation. Unlike quantitative studies in which a researcher interprets data with measures of statistical significance, qualitative data are narrowed and thematically categorized through the lens of the researcher or research team. Participants in qualitative studies may be concerned about being misrepresented when data are interpreted. It is the researcher's ethical responsibility to analyze and interpret qualitative data using best practices for trustworthiness. The study design should include reflexivity and periodic member checking for the most appropriate representation of the data collected.

Another ethical issue in qualitative research is reporting and disseminating findings. The researcher must inform study participants about ways in which research reports will be distributed, and the target audiences who will receive the findings. The research finding should always be summarized and provided to the participants in a way most relevant to them.

These ethical issues related to qualitative research can be addressed through engagement with stakeholders, key informants, and members of the sample population in all phases of the research process. Community-based participatory research (CBPR) is one example of a collaborative approach to research that facilitates engagement of participants throughout a study. In-depth knowledge of the community though collaborative approaches can help during planning (e.g., making sure questions are relevant), implementing (e.g., learning ways to reduce participant burden), and disseminating qualitative research (e.g., making sure interpretation accurately represents the qualitative data).

In summary, an ethical approach to qualitative studies includes

- engagement of participants throughout the process,
- knowledge of the topic and the community,

- cultural competency of the research team,
- confidentiality of data,
- reduced participant burden,
- use of detailed informed consent forms tailored to the population, and
- accurate interpretation and reporting.

CHAPTER DISCUSSION QUESTIONS

1. Describe a way in which you might engage a participant sample for a qualitative study using interviews with teen fathers to gain insight on the experience of being a teen father.
2. What are some ethical advantages to qualitative research over quantitative research?
3. How could you convince a proponent of quantitative research on the merits of qualitative research?
4. Describe ways you could ensure rigor in a qualitative study of cyberbullying.

RESEARCH PROJECT CHECK-IN

Are You Conducting a Qualitative Study?

Qualitative research provides unique perspectives on public health issues, but the research can be complex. If you are conducting qualitative research as part of your class project, carefully consider the qualitative approach to your study. Plan for high-quality study design and record what you plan to do in order to implement the best study possible. Also, keep in mind the additional ethical considerations of this type of research such as sampling, confidentiality, and participant burden. Make sure you have knowledge of your target population and tailor your study to its characteristics, culture, or climate if needed.

PUBLIC HEALTH RESEARCH METHODS IN REAL LIFE

The Sum of the Parts

Davian was new to the concept of qualitative research. He was an epidemiologist and conducted a few disease case studies, but mostly worked with numbers neatly organized in two-by-two tables. Now he was part of an academic research team funded to conduct a comprehensive evaluation of a large urban park. The park was a free community resource for health-enhancing outdoor activity. Park administration wanted the evaluation to inform strategic planning and fuel enhanced financial support from city officials. They were interested in who uses the park and what they do when visiting the park. They were also interested in who does not use the park. City officials hypothesized that many people living in lower income communities adjacent to the park did not visit it as much as residents of other communities. If this was true, the city wanted strategies to address this issue incorporated into the park's strategic plan. The evaluation was on a tight timeline due to the timing of strategic planning and municipal fiscal appropriations.

Davian was excited to be a part of the surveillance team. He helped develop the ways in which to capture use of the many park amenities such as trails, bike paths, sports fields, and picnic areas. His epidemiological background came in handy as he created a detailed surveillance plan using observation, technology, and surveys. Two other team members were planning some qualitative work to supplement the quantitative data being collected.

A few months into the project, a key research team member left to pursue a dream job in another state. It was too late to hire someone else due to the tight timeline, but there was now a gap in people to work on the qualitative component of the evaluation. The leader of the research team asked Davian if he would work on the qualitative part of the evaluation since the quantitative surveillance was going well. He mentioned the benefits of being skilled in both quantitative and qualitative methods, and this experience would be good for his career. Besides, he would not be alone in this work, as there was one other team member doing the qualitative work.

Davian accepted the challenge with trepidation. To ease his uncertainty, he had lengthy conversations with a few of his mentors who specialized in qualitative methods. He also read several qualitative studies published on topics similar to their evaluation. Even after his research, he was still unsure about the rigor and value of qualitative data for the park evaluation. He was a numbers person and analyzing words seemed very subjective. He wondered how they would come up with significant findings without p values! He also wondered how input from a few interviews or focus groups could represent the thousands of people who live in the communities around the park.

His research partner helped ease his concerns. She explained to him the careful planning that went into sampling and recruitment. They had community members on the evaluation advisory board who provided guidance on how to make the data collection relevant to participants while still facilitating achievement of the goals of the evaluation. They would start with interviewing key stakeholders, then conduct focus groups in conjunction with local community meetings. They also had a plan to interview parents of students in a school near the park. This multilevel strategy would provide a broad scope of insight. They would adhere to best practices of qualitative research, and be sure to use member-checking as a way to add credibility to the results. When she explained how they track every step in the research process and employ key strategies for improving reliability in analysis, Davian felt more at ease. There was even computer software to help organize and analyze data.

After a few meetings with the research team, Davian felt more confident that he could contribute to the qualitative components of the evaluation. He even felt eager to begin interviewing the stakeholders. He realized that focused expertise in one research methodology is fine for something, but for many complex public health issues, a more comprehensive approach is needed. And numbers will not add up to the whole story.

Critical Thinking Questions

1. How would you convince someone of the merits of qualitative research in public health?
2. Reflexivity in qualitative research is vital to the process. How could someone new to qualitative work (like Davian) gain an understanding of and skills in this concept?
3. If you were Davian, what other ways would you prepare for conducting qualitative data collection?
4. What other ways could the evaluation team enhance credibility of the qualitative component of the park evaluation?
5. If you were Davian's qualitative coworker, what would you tell him about ethical issues related to collecting qualitative data, especially from vulnerable populations?

COUNCIL ON EDUCATION FOR PUBLIC HEALTH FOUNDATIONAL KNOWLEDGE AND COMPETENCIES

Foundational Knowledge

Profession and Science of Public Health

- Explain the critical importance of evidence in advancing public health knowledge.
- Explain the role of quantitative and qualitative methods and sciences in describing and assessing a population's health.

Evidence-Based Approaches to Public Health

- Select quantitative and qualitative data-collection methods appropriate for a given public health context.

Planning and Management to Promote Health

- Assess population needs, assets, and capacities that affect communities' health.
- Apply awareness of cultural values and practices to the design or implementation of public health policies or programs.

REFERENCES

1. Flick U. In: *An introduction to Qualitative Research*. 6th ed. Thousand Oaks, CA: Sage; 2018:5–10.

2. Bailey L. The origin and success of qualitative research. *Int J Mark Res*. 2014;56(2):167–183. doi:10.2501/IJMR-2014-013

3. DiSantis KI, Grier SA, Odoms-Young A, et al. What "price" means when buying food: insights from a multisite qualitative study with black Americans. *Am J Public Health*. 2013;103(3):516–522. doi:10.2105/AJPH.2012.301149

4. He M, Wilmoth S, Bustos D, et al. Latino church leader's perspectives on childhood obesity prevention. *Am J Prev Med*. 2013;44(3 suppl 3):s232–s239. doi:10.1016/j.amepre.2012.11.014

5. Kegler MC, Anderson K, Bundy LT, et al. A qualitative study about creating smoke-free home rules in American Indian and Alaska native households. *J Community Health*. 2019;44(4):684–693. doi:10.1007/s10900-019-00666-1

6. Sledge JA, Jensen CE, Cibulka NJ, et al. The male voice: a qualitative assessment of young men's communication preferences about HPV and 9v HPV. *J Community Health*. 2019;44(5):998–1008. doi:10.1007/s10900-019-00674-1

7. Gilbert AS, Duncan DD, Beck AM, et al. A qualitative study identifying barriers and facilitators of physical activity in rural communities. *J Environ Public Health*. 2019;Article ID 7298692. doi:10.1155/2019/7298692

8. Nowak CG, Sheedy K, Bursey K, et al. Promoting influenza vaccination: insights from a qualitative meta-analysis of 14 years of influenza-related communications research by US centers for disease control. *Vaccine*. 2015;33(4):2741–2756. doi:10.1016/j.vaccine.2015.04.064

9. Cochrane Collaborative. 20 qualitative research and Cochrane reviews. Cochrane handbook for systematic reviews of interventions, Version 5. 2011. Accessed October 9, 2019. https://handbook-5-1.cochrane.org/chapter_20/20_qualitative_research_and_cochrane_reviews.htm

10. Hansen H, Holmes S, Lindemann D. Ethnography of health for social change: impact on public perception and policy. *Soc Sci Med*. 2013;99:116–118. doi:10.1016/j.socscimed.2013.11.001

11. Corbin JM, Strauss AL. *Basics of Qualitative Research: Techniques and Procedures for Developing Grounded Theory*. 4th ed. Sage Publications; 2014. Accessed January 22, 2019. https://us.sagepub.com/en-us/nam/basics-of-qualitative-research/book235578

12. Yin RK. *Case Study Research: Design and Methods*. 5th ed. Thousand Oaks, CA: Sage; 2014.

13. Community Preventive Services Task Force. Interventions to increase active travel to school. Guide to community preventive services. 2018. Accessed October 9, 2019. https://www.thecommunityguide.org/content/interventions-increase-active-travel-school. Published 2018

14. Eyler AA, Brownson RC, Doescher MP, et al. Policies related to active transport to and from school: a multisite case study. *Health Educ Res*. 2007;23(6):963–975. doi:10.1093/her/cym061

15. Guba E, Lincoln Y. Competing paradigms in qualitative research. In: Denzin N, Lincoln Y, eds. *Handbook of Qualitative Research*. Thousand Oaks, CA: Sage Publications; 1994:105–117.

16. Jones E, Eyler AA, Nguyen L, et al. It's all in the lens: differences in views on obesity prevention between advocates and policy makers. *Child Obes*. 2012;8(3):243–250. doi:10.1089/chi.2011.0038

17. Eyler AA, Vest JR. Environmental and policy factors related to physical activity in rural white women. *Women Health*. 2002;36(2):109–119. doi:10.1300/J013v36n02_08

ADDITIONAL READINGS AND RESOURCES

Corbin J, Strauss A. *Basics of Qualitative Research*. 4th ed. Thousand Oaks, CA: Sage; 2015.

Higgins JPT, Thomas J, Chandler J, et al., eds. Critical appraisal of qualitative research. In: *Cochrane Handbook for Systematic Reviews of Interventions*. Version 6.0. Cochrane; 2019 [chapter 4]. https://training.cochrane.org/cochrane-handbook-systematic-reviews-interventions

Wolff B, Mahoney F, Lohiniva, et al. Collecting and analyzing qualitative data. In: *The CDC Field Epidemiology Manual*. Atlanta GA: Centers for Disease Control and Prevention; 2018. https://www.cdc.gov/eis/field-epi-manual/chapters/Qualitative-Data.html

Trotter TR. Qualitative research sample design and sample size. Resolving and unresolved issues for inferential imperatives. *Prev Med*. 2012;55:398–400. doi:10.1016/j.ypmed.2012.07.003

Qualitative Data Collection

Always bring two tape recorders to interviews.
—Jonathon Small, writer/editor

LEARNING OBJECTIVES

The reader will be able to

- Describe the main methods of qualitative data collection.
- Explain the impact of technology on qualitative data collection.
- Describe best practices for qualitative data collection.

INTRODUCTION

Qualitative data collection is based on very detailed information gathered from people who know about the topic of interest, and through observation of settings and interactions. The data could be a record of complex thoughts, feelings, behaviors, and interactions of participants. Qualitative data can also be a documentation of what is observed in the environment. Unlike quantitative data measured in exact quantities or used to determine causal relationships, qualitative data is meant to be a source for an interpretive approach. These data provide rich and detailed information for exploring and understanding public health issues.

Qualitative data can be collected at one point in time, or the research design may include using multiple time points. To gain an understanding of how a phenomenon, process, or perspective changes over time, the time series approach is useful. This approach is particularly useful for studying health behaviors. Suppose you wanted to study social support and weight loss in women. You might collect qualitative data at the beginning and end of an intervention. Identifying perceptions of social support as healthy eating behaviors evolve could provide useful evidence for tailoring future interventions.

There are several common ways to qualitatively collect data. Each process has benefits and limitations, and the researcher should carefully consider these when selecting methods for data collection. The methods described in this chapter include individual and group interviewing, observation, gathering content (e.g., documents) for qualitative content analysis, and collaborative approaches.

INDIVIDUAL AND GROUP INTERVIEWING

Interviews, conducted individually or in groups, are a common qualitative data-collection strategy used in public health research. Through interviews, researchers can gain broad and meaningful insight into the participant's perspective. Unlike quantitative surveys, interviewing allows the researcher to clarify the questions for the participant if needed, as well as probe deeper into their responses. This helps to capture more in-depth and accurate data. Interviewing allows for a certain degree of flexibility in how an inquiry is administered. Issues may come up during interviews that were not originally considered, but still relevant to the topic of interest. Interview flexibility facilitates further exploration of these factors. Suppose you are interviewing older adults on perceptions of safety in their neighborhood. Several people you interview mention the fact that seeing one specific person walking their dog makes the person feel safe. You could explore this finding in more detail to figure out why this one factor increased participant's perception.

The qualitative-methodology literature identifies many different ways to categorize types of interviews. In general, interviews can be informal, semistructured (i.e., guided), or structured. **Informal interviews** are impromptu conversations typically taking place within field research and matched with observational data. There are no predetermined questions in these interviews, and the process flows and stops as needed. In **semistructured interviews**, the researcher is guided by some structure or format. A semi-structured interview is a hybrid of a conversational approach and a more structured interview. Semistructured interviews are conducted using a list of broad and open-ended questions, but with some adaptability in obtaining the information from the participant. **Structured interviews** are the least flexible of the three types. In structured interviews, the researcher uses a detailed interview guide to ensure all participants are asked the same questions. A structured guide also improves consistency across multiple interviewers. More structure reduces the potential of interviewer bias, and variability in way the interviews may be conducted. Public health researchers should consider the research topic, characteristics of the population and setting, as well as the overall research question when selecting the most appropriate type of interview.

Whatever type of interview you choose, there are general qualities of interviewees that could improve the outcome of this qualitative research method. First, participants need to have the necessary information on the topic of interest. If you wanted to study the perception of an infant sleep-health media campaign, you would interview people who are aware of the campaign. It would be quite a short interview if participants did not know the campaign existed! Participants also need to be motivated to share information with you. Some people may be more likely than others to agree to be interviewed, and then actually provide meaningful information. Using information from past studies, doing formative work, and getting to know the population prior to interviews will help in selecting people with whom to talk. People you wish to interview also need to be able to clearly understand the questions. Literacy and culture can influence how well participants realize what is being asked. Preparation by the researcher and pilot testing are needed to create meaningful data from the interaction.

"That is not what we call it."

When pilot-testing interview questions for a study on fee policies charged for high school sports, Eyler and colleagues learned that the term "pay to play" was not used by athletic directors to describe these policies. Those involved in the pilot shared that "pay to play" implies that if students pay a fee, they will be guaranteed to actually play in the games. The athletic directors used the terms "pay to participate" or "sports participation fees" to clarify that the fees would not guarantee that the students would play in the games. The interview guide and subsequent surveys were changed to reflect this new information.[16]

Interviews can also be planned with people who have specialized expertise or knowledge about the topic or problem being studied. **Key-informant interviews** aim to gather expert opinions from people who have a higher level of knowledge about the topic than those directly impacted by the issue of study. For example, church leaders could serve as key informants in a study of a faith-based diabetes intervention. School administrators might be key informants for research on policies relating to students' possession of electronic cigarettes. Data from key-informant interviews can be a sole source of research data, paired with other interview data, or matched with quantitative resources to help explain a complex public health topic. For instance, data from the key-informant school administrators in the previous example could be supplemented with student interviews, and/or prevalence of policy infraction.

Interviews can take place via telephone, face-to-face, or even online using visual-conferencing technologies. Telephone interviews are convenient, do not require travel to interview sites, and are low cost. Participants can talk with the researcher in a private setting of their choosing. However, this method lacks the face-to-face contact of in-person interviews. Without personal trust or rapport, the participant may be less likely to agree to have the conversation recorded. In addition, it is impossible to assess body language or nonverbal cues over the telephone. In-person interviews have the benefit of personal interaction, but may be more of a logistical challenge. They should be conducted in a quiet and comfortable space convenient for the participant. The researcher should provide transportation and childcare if needed. Online conversation applications (e.g., Skype, Google Hangout, FaceTime, Zoom) can also be used for conducting interviews. These platforms combine the convenience of telephone interviewing with a form of face-to face contact via video. As technology improves and these applications become mainstream, utility for qualitative research will increase. However, participants need a smartphone or computer device, internet or data connection, and familiarity with technology. This can be a barrier to participation for some groups. Technological difficulties can also happen. Researchers using online methods should be prepared for troubleshooting.

All modes of collecting interview data require proper planning. Once participants agree to be interviewed, a convenient date and time needs to be established. The researcher must communicate a confirmation and send reminders to participants. Even with the most diligent preparation, interviews may not go as planned and will need to be rescheduled. Be sure to build in extra time for potential data-collection delays.

Keeping a record of what is said during interviews is a key aspect of data collection. Even with diligent note taking, specific details of the conversation or context may be difficult to remember. Also, constant note-taking can be distracting, especially in face-to-face interviews. Audio recording is an option to document what was said; it also enhances reliability and clarity in analysis. Consent documents must clearly include provisions for recording conversations, and the extent to which the identity of participants will be used in analysis and reporting.

Many options for quality, inexpensive digital recorders are widely available. Most models have the capability to easily download recordings to computer files, which can be transcribed and used in analysis. Audio recording, however, is not foolproof. Background noise can make conversations difficult to hear during playback. Also, expert interviewers recommend always using a backup recorder. Devices can break, stop working, or batteries can die. It would be a definite setback if part or all of a conversation was not captured. Best practices include using a recorder (or two), taking supplementary notes, and debriefing with the research team to ensure capture of comprehensive and quality interview data.

FOCUS GROUPS

Focus groups are like group interviews. Guided by a moderator, a group of people discuss the topic of interest. Because more than one person provides input, focus groups are a good way to get varied opinions about an issue. Group dynamics and social interactions among the participants emerge in focus groups, and can enhance the discussion. One person may say something that invokes a response from someone else in the group, and the depth of the conversation builds. Noting how meaning emerges within conversations can be useful to add to analysis. See Table 12.1 for ways to analyze the interactions within focus groups. In some ways, focus groups can be less intimidating for participants than one-on-one interviews. The presence of others mitigates the potential power differential between researcher and participant in the group.[1]

The decision to use focus groups to collect qualitative data should be based on several factors. First, consider the research topic. Think about whether people would feel comfortable sharing information about the topic in front of others. Gaining insight about perceptions of a media campaign may be more easily discussed in a group setting than a more personal topic such as birth control practices. Second, consider the target population. Focus group success relies on participants being comfortable with one another. Characteristics of the target population may impact comfort level and group dynamics. For example, in a focus group about physical activity, women who are marathon runners might intimidate women who are sedentary. Sometimes researchers may conduct separate groups if this aligns with the research goal. Perhaps one group with sedentary women and another with elite athletes would be warranted. Third, the moderator matters. A researcher planning focus groups should have access to a skilled moderator who is familiar with the topic and the target population. Matching moderator characteristics with group characteristics may be important in certain studies. For instance, women may be more likely to openly talk about birth control practices with a moderator who is a woman. It is a good idea to refer to the literature on studies with similar populations to gain insight on lessons learned from previous research. See Table 12.2 for examples of how focus groups have been used in public health research.

TABLE 12.1 INTERACTION AS A COMPONENT OF FOCUS GROUP DATA ANALYSIS

Group Component	Interaction Question
Members	• How did members react to responses from certain individuals? • Was a particular member encouraged or silenced? • Were alliances formed?
Topics	• What topics produced consensus? • What questions resulted in response disagreement? • What common experiences were expressed? • Did the group collectively come up with new insights on the topic?
Process	• What nonverbal signs were used during discussion? • How did members react to the flow of the questions? • How well did members adhere to the topic of interest?

Source: Data from Willis K, Green J, Daly J, et al. Perils and possibilities: achieving best evidence from focus groups in public health research. *Aust NZ J Public Health.* 2009;33(2):131–136.[2]

TABLE 12.2 EXAMPLES OF FOCUS GROUP RESEARCH IN PUBLIC HEALTH

Citation	Purpose/Aim	Sample
Chan et al.[3]	The purpose of this exploratory study is to understand how women respond to examples of physical activity promotion messages.	40 women, stratified by race/ethnicity and levels of physical activity Eight focus groups conducted
Brown et al.[4]	The purpose of the study was to conduct focus groups with Mexican Americans in an impoverished rural community on the Texas–Mexico border to identify current barriers to adopting healthier lifestyles and to obtain recommendations for diabetes prevention.	Three groups with seven to 12 participants ($N = 27$) All were individuals diagnosed with type 2 diabetes or prediabetes
Camenga et al.[5]	This study describes middle, high school, and college students' beliefs about, and experiences with e-cigarettes for cigarette-smoking cessation.	18 groups ($N = 127$) of male and female smokers

(continued)

Citation	Purpose/Aim	Sample
TABLE 12.2 EXAMPLES OF FOCUS GROUP RESEARCH IN PUBLIC HEALTH *(continued)*		
Cohen et al.[6]	This study examined the acceptability and impact of a primary care–based informational intervention on facilitators and barriers to use of the statewide SNAP incentive program Double Up Food Bucks.	Five groups (*N* = 26) with a purposive sample of SNAP-enrolled adults from a Michigan clinic serving low-income patients
Griffith et al.[7]	This study explored how African American men define *manhood* and *health*, and implications of these definitions for health behavior and health outcomes.	7 focus groups with 73 African American men aged 24–77

SNAP, Supplemental Nutrition Assistance Program.

Several factors facilitate successful implementation of focus groups. Size of the group is an important factor. There is some disparity in the literature on recommended group size, but according to Krueger and Casey, five to 10 per group is best, with six to eight being optimal.[8] The group should include enough people to facilitate easy engagement in the discussion, but not so large the discussion becomes unmanageable. In groups that are too large, participants may be more likely to start smaller side conversations, which can be distracting and dilute the focus group process. When planning focus groups, always assume that not everyone will show up. Researchers often need to over-recruit participants to achieve the optimal focus group size.

Focus groups can be an efficient way to collect qualitative data from several people at once, but only if the conversation is well facilitated. Personality types of participants can clash; a shy person may not want to speak up if another group member dominates the conversation. A good moderator finds ways to engage all participants by asking questions such as "Who else has another way of looking at the issue?" or by asking each person to take turns responding to a question. A good moderator can also encourage discussion when no one initiates conversation. Pausing with silence, then clarifying the question or probing for more information can help facilitate sharing. Focus group conversations can get off track, too. It is the moderator's job to minimize discussions not related to the main research purpose.

Note-taking is also an important part of capturing focus group data. A member of the research team (not the moderator) should take notes during the discussion. The note-taker can record things not picked up by an audio recording, such as nonverbal reactions of participants. A conversation may seem to be flowing smoothly, but noted frowns and crossed arms of participants may indicate otherwise. Noteworthy quotes or revelations can also be recorded. These quotes can be used in analysis to exemplify important concepts. Notes may also reveal a view of context aside from that of the moderator. The note-taker and moderator should debrief immediately after the event to share notes and thoughts about the process.

DEVELOPING QUESTIONS FOR INTERVIEWS AND FOCUS GROUPS

Well-developed qualitative questions can yield valuable research information. Most interview and focus group questions are open-ended, allowing the participants to answer more freely than if response options were provided. This results in rich, detailed data that is the hallmark of qualitative research. The first step in developing good questions is to decide what information is needed to achieve the aims of the research. Ask yourself:

- Why do I want this information?
- How does this information relate to my research question?
- How does this information relate to my overall analysis and dissemination plans?

Although your initial list of interesting things to ask may be broad, doing this self-reflection helps focus the questions on the most important information needs.

As you develop questions, maintain connection to the characteristics of the target population. Consider culture, literacy, and ethics when crafting the questions. Clarity and simplicity should be balanced with relevance and appropriateness. Visual activities, such as photo-sorting, and vignettes can supplement questions and make concepts easier to understand. These methods also help when there are varying levels of understanding or literacy among members of the group. Pilot test questions with a few members of your target population to be sure the wording matches the perception of the group. If the questions do not result in the desired information, reformulate them and pilot test again.

PHOTO-SORTING AS A QUALITATIVE DATA TOOL

In order to increase local participation in a community's Open Streets event, researchers elicited input through focus groups with parents and adolescents who were residents in a nearby neighborhood. Participants were given a stack of pictures of people doing a range of activities and asked to choose the top three they would participate in, and the top three their family would enjoy. After the sorting exercise, the moderator facilitated a discussion about activity preferences. This information was useful in prioritizing and planning event activities, and kept the participants engaged during the inquiry.[17]

You want the interview or focus group questions to elicit the most information possible, so avoid using questions that can be answered with a yes/no response. Participants may respond yes/no and nothing more. Asking, *"Do you take breaks during your typical workday?"* can be answered yes or no, and requires prompting for follow-up. A better inquiry would be *"Describe your typical workday."* Wording questions in a way that requires a more detailed and thoughtful response results in better qualitative data.

The flexibility of the qualitative research process allows for the addition of **probes**, or optional prompts to elicit follow-up information. Probes can be used to get more details about what a participant said (e.g., *Tell me more about that* . . .) or for clarification (e.g., *It sounds like you are saying* . . .). Probes can be follow-up questions when the participant only provides a partial answer. Suppose you are interested in learning about public health issues stimulating personal interest in public health practice. A question and probes might be:

Question: What made you become interested in public health as a profession?

Probes: What populations were of concern to you?

What health conditions were of interest?

Probes are used at the discretion of the interviewer or moderator. You may not need to ask the follow-up probes if the participant provides an answer with enough details. However, sometimes participants need time to think about how to respond. Silence itself can be a probe. Allowing time for a participant to think for a moment before answering may result in a more thorough answer.

Once the questions are developed and pilot tested, you need to plan their order and flow. The beginning of the interview sets the tone for the discussion.[9] After obtaining informed consent, explaining the research goals, and giving the introduction, start with a "warm-up" question. This can help build rapport and is a good way to ease into the rest of the interview. Next, think about the logical flow of the questions. Responses from one question might inform how others are asked. Order the questions to accommodate this progression. Qualitative research experts recommend sequencing the questions from general to specific.[8] Personal stories are a good way to end an interview or focus group discussion. In an interview on barriers to healthy eating, a final inquiry might be, *"Tell me a story about an experience you had buying healthy food at the store."* Another example might be, *"Tell me a story about a time you made a healthy meal."* These stories allow participants to elaborate on their own experience in an unstructured way. Story-driven anecdotes are powerful pieces of qualitative data. You also might ask the participants to reflect on the previous discussion in a way that encourages them to highlight their perceptions about the most important issues. An example could be, *"Suppose you had 1 minute to talk to the mayor about the need for healthy food access in your neighborhood. What would you say?"* The last question should provide some closure for the interview and leave the participants satisfied with their input.

USING OBSERVATION TO COLLECT QUALITATIVE DATA

Observing people, events, or environments is another way to gather qualitative data. Systematic observation (as described in Chapter 9, Quantitative Data Collection) may be used as a quantitative data-collection method, but observation can also be less structured. Instead of counts or measures, qualitative observation is built on detailed descriptions and narratives of natural settings. Rooted in anthropological studies, observational approaches are common in public health research. See Table 12.3 for examples of how qualitative observational methodology may be used in varied public health studies.

There are two main parameters outlining categories of observational research. The first is participation. **Participant observation** occurs when the researcher becomes a participant in the group or setting during observation. In **nonparticipant observation,** the researcher observes the group or setting without taking part. In both types, the researcher can choose whether to disclose their role as an observer or remain discreet. Participants' knowledge of an observation may bias results, as seen in the Hawthorne experiments (see Chapter 9, Quantitative Data Collection). **Direct observation** occurs when the researcher observes

TABLE 12.3 EXAMPLES OF QUALITATIVE OBSERVATION IN PUBLIC HEALTH RESEARCH

Topic	Observation Examples
Physical activity and social support	• Social activity in public spaces such as parks or sidewalks • Children's interactions with one another in sports or on playground
Nutrition	• The checkout at a grocery store • Interaction between fast-food cashier and patron
Chronic disease	• Sunscreen behaviors at beaches or outdoor spaces • Smoking behavior in designated smoking areas
Environmental health	• Disposal of litter at outdoor events • Use of refillable water bottle stations in public spaces
Healthcare	• Interactions between healthcare practitioner and patient

behaviors or interactions as they occur; for example, observing elementary school children on a playground during recess. **Indirect observation** is the process of observing the effects or results of behaviors or interactions. In a preschool setting, indirect observation might be used to collect information on how children use free playtime. The researcher can observe the play space after the children leave to see what toys were used and how items were left. Researchers should choose the type of observation based on their research topic, research goals, target population, and ethical considerations.

As discussed in Chapter 9, Quantitative Data Collection, technological advancements have increased the opportunities for observation as a research method. Researchers can do the observing themselves in real time (i.e., human observation), or utilize mechanical observation. In mechanical observation, a device (e.g., security camera) captures the observation. These devices record images for analysis after the behavior or interaction occurs.

There are several advantages to using observation in research. First, this method does not rely on people providing information. The researcher can see what people do instead of relying on self-reports. Also, observation techniques allow collecting data at a time and place when the behavior or interaction is occurring. Mechanical observation increases reliability by making recorded images available to more than one observer to confirm data. Observation can be a powerful qualitative data-collection method, but it has limitations. Subjectivity and bias of the observer may influence what is recorded. Therefore it is critical to train observers in the difference between observations versus interpretation. Suppose a researcher is observing a classroom setting and records the room is hot. "Hot" is a subjective interpretation of the temperature in the room. What feels hot to one person, might feel cool to another person. If temperature is important to record, the observer should record the actual number from the thermometer. Another limitation on observation is it is only a "snapshot" of a point in time. Multiple observations or triangulating with other data sources can broaden the scope of what is being studied. Observing behaviors or interactions does not allow the researcher to take into account any underlying motives, attitudes, or internal conditions of the situation. Researchers should determine the utility of observational methods based on their research topic and overall research goals.

DATA COLLECTION FOR QUALITATIVE CONTENT ANALYSIS

Content analysis is a research strategy used to determine the presence of concepts and themes with text or recorded information. This method can be quantitative (e.g., word counts) or qualitative. Examples of materials used in content analysis include policies, transcribed speeches, meeting minutes, videos, and media articles. There are many online sources for content analysis such as blogs, social media posts, and reviews. This method can be quantitative (e.g., counting words and phrases) or qualitative, for which the researcher thematically summarizes and interprets the text to make observable and reproducible inferences.[10] According to Krippendorff,[10] the content analysis process must address the following:

1. Which data are analyzed?
2. How are they defined?
3. What is the population from which they are drawn?
4. What is the context relative to which the data are analyzed?
5. What are the boundaries for the analysis?
6. What is the target of the inferences?

Similar to other research methods, content analysis starts with a research question and sampling plan.

Examples

Research question: How is the connection between diet and breast cancer portrayed in magazines geared toward women?
Sampling plan: Collect articles about breast cancer from the top-10 best-selling women's magazines from the past 3 years.

Research question: To what extent are disciplines outside of public health included in state health department strategic plans?
Sampling plan: Collect current strategic plans from all state health departments.

Research question: How has the presentation of the topic of birth control changed in prime-time television over the past 50 years?
Sampling plan: Choose the top 10 television shows for each year. Develop a selection method for representation of shows over time.

One benefit of doing qualitative content analysis (similar to observations) is the data are not collected directly from people. Also, access to many sources of data is relatively easy and inexpensive, especially for resources that are online. Multiple researchers and computer-aided analysis helps reduce bias and subjectivity in content analysis. One disadvantage is the analysis only offers surface-level interpretation and lacks deeper meaning or explanation of emergent themes. However, it can be used as a catalyst for more in-depth future research studies. Content analysis may also be limited by missing or incomplete documents. Researchers planning to use content analysis should carefully consider potential issues related to information access and continuity.

COMMUNITY-BASED PARTICIPATORY RESEARCH

Community-based participatory research (CBPR) is a community engagement model that involves community partners in all aspects of the research process.[11] It is a way to encourage empowerment and social change within communities. The basis of CBPR is shared experiences, perspectives, and decision-making. CBPR includes many opportunities to gather qualitative data, and can produce multiple and varied perspectives throughout the research process. The use of qualitative methods in CBPR can produce deep insight into public health issues. The quality and depth of the data are enhanced by the mutual respect that develops between the researcher and the community through the research process.

In addition to interviews and focus groups, other qualitative data-collection methods are commonly used in CBPR or other collaborative approaches. Because whole communities are often the focus of study, researchers can use several types of group information-gathering approaches. **Use of community forums** (e.g., town hall meetings) is one strategy for gathering qualitative data. These are open meetings where members of the community come together to discuss an issue of common concern. Discussion can reveal diverse perspectives from a broad audience. As in focus group research, the interactions among attendees provide additional insight into the issue. A more structured group information-gathering approach is a **listening session**. Using predetermined questions, a facilitator guides the listening session discussion. Listening sessions commonly include perspectives of invited speakers, panels, or opinion leaders. Both community forums and listening sessions can be observed using qualitative methodologies. The conversations can also be recorded and transcribed for qualitative data analysis.

Driving in or walking around a community can provide valuable qualitative data. Windshield tours (observations from a moving vehicle) and walking surveys (observations on foot) can help to document specific factors difficult to assess in other ways. Some studies include community partners in these tours to gain their insight, but also to broaden the perspective of the researcher. Windshield tours or walking surveys elucidate community assets, challenges, and qualities useful to a comprehensive community research study.

Text and observations are not the only data that can be collected in collaborative research approaches. **Photovoice** is a visual research methodology in which participants (instead of researchers) collect the data. It is sometimes referred to as photo elicitation. In this approach, participants are given cameras to help them document and communicate about the topic of interest. Photovoice enables people to record and reflect their community's strengths and concerns, and promotes discussion about the issues documented in the photos.[12] Photovoice is particularly relevant to research with vulnerable populations or groups without the capacity to provide input in other ways. First documented as a data-collection strategy decades ago, photovoice is now a powerful qualitative approach to research. Examples of photovoice in public health research include topics such as children's perception of healthy environments,[13] adult disease management,[14] and experiences of people with disabilities.[15] A literature database search of the term "photovoice" will reveal the broad application of this method in public health.

Tips for Collecting Qualitative Data

1. Make sure the collection method is appropriate for the target population.
2. Take time to develop and pilot test questions.
3. Get trained in interviewing or facilitation.
4. Be an active listener and observer.
5. Be sensitive to the human experience of sharing information.

CHAPTER DISCUSSION QUESTIONS

1. Compare and contrast using individual interviews versus focus groups for a research project on stress and spousal caregiving for adults with cognitive impairment.
2. Why is it important to pilot test interview questions?
3. What are examples of public health research topics that would be well suited for qualitative observation?
4. What are ways to use content analysis in a study of media coverage of emergency preparedness?

RESEARCH PROJECT CHECK-IN

Dig Deep

Qualitative data collection digs deep into public health issues. Before choosing your method of data collection, look at past studies to get a sense of best practices for your topic and population. Think about the ethical considerations such as consent and confidentiality. If you are using interviews or focus groups, develop your questions with your main research question or study aim in mind. Just as in qualitative surveys and data collection, it is critical to pilot test the questions or instruments within the population or setting of interest. Also, do not underestimate the potential for equipment failures or technological difficulties—especially digital recorders!

PUBLIC HEALTH RESEARCH METHODS IN REAL LIFE

Not in Front of Everybody

There is sometimes a gap in what people say they do, and what they actually do. This is a common concern in public health studies. Participants may alter what they report due to their perception of what others (including the researcher) might think. The risk of social desirability bias can be even greater in settings where peers are present, especially when the health topic is a sensitive one. Flora learned this the hard way. She was an employee health consultant hired to explore ways to improve healthy eating in employees of a company that processed warrantees for home appliances. There were about 100 employees, mostly women.

Flora's research plan included some formative data collection through focus groups. She developed a moderator's guide using questions from similar studies. Flora and her assistant recruited 16 volunteers to participate, and divided them into two groups. She made sure she had good representation from all the departments. Because she did not want management presence to influence what the participants said, she did not include them in the groups. The two focus group meetings were held back-to-back during the workday.

Flora asked the participants to describe the food they eat during the typical workday. Several people in the first focus group mentioned how they always bring food from home to eat at work. Other participants agreed with this statement and also reported the benefits of meal planning. When one person mentioned the vending machines located in the break room, there were lots of comments about the unhealthy choices in them. When asked about their vending purchases, no one spoke up. One person finally spoke up and said they never buy things from the vending machine and would "rather eat the crumbs in my keyboard" if they were starving. Other comments were similar. From information given by this group, Flora noted the vending machines were rarely used as a source of food for the employees. Participants in the second focus group provided information consistent with the first group. Almost everyone reported bringing food and snacks from home to eat during the workday.

Flora supplemented the focus group information with other data to get a full understanding of the company environment and culture. During the food environment audit at the worksite, she noticed the vending machines were nearly empty. Just as she was counting items in the machines, a representative from the vending company came to refill them. Flora explained the purpose of the audit to the vending rep and asked whether she could acquire sales data for the machines in the break room. He wrote down a number for her to call to get the data. As he handed her the number, he told her he comes to this site at least twice a week to restock the machines. This comment made her question the truth in what was said in the focus groups.

Flora decided to mention this discrepancy to the human resources (HR) manager who hired her as a consultant. When the HR manager reviewed the list of focus group participants, she immediately spotted it. Each group included a company "wellness champion." These champions were volunteers who were supposed to motivate employees to be healthier and act as liaisons to wellness resources. The champions were sometimes called "health sergeants" by the rest of the employees. It became clear to Flora that focus group participants were influenced by the presence of the wellness champions and did not want to admit unhealthy eating; specifically, purchasing junk food from the vending machines.

When Flora conducted follow-up interviews one-on-one with employees, she gained insight into their eating behaviors. The most common barriers to healthy eating by employees were long work hours, lack of formal lunch breaks, and no refrigerator for storing food brought from home. Many of them also reported lack of confidence in company management to make the eating situation better. A few employees talked about how company management promoted wellness champions as a health-promotion program, when in fact, they were having a negative effect.

Flora analyzed the interview data and wrote a report for the company administration. They worked together to use the qualitative information to develop a survey on perceptions, priorities, and recommendations for improving healthy eating among employees. Although it is impossible to know everything about a research population, Flora realized she could have done a better job in planning the qualitative data collection if she knew more about the organization and included the employees in the process from the very beginning.

Critical Thinking Questions

1. What preparation should have taken place before Flora planned and implemented the focus groups?
2. What should Flora do with the data from the focus group? Even though it became apparent that there was social desirability bias, is the data worth analyzing? Why or why not?
3. How could a researcher test their topics of interest for the potential of social desirability?
4. Flora just happened to realize the bias when collecting audit data. How might have biased results impacted the outcome, especially recommendations back to company management?
5. What characteristics of a workplace might make employees more prone to social desirability?

COUNCIL ON EDUCATION FOR PUBLIC HEALTH FOUNDATIONAL KNOWLEDGE AND COMPETENCIES

Foundational Knowledge
Profession and Science of Public Health
- Explain the critical importance of evidence in advancing public health knowledge.
- Explain the role of quantitative and qualitative methods and sciences in describing and assessing a population's health.

Evidence-Based Approaches to Public Health
- Select quantitative and qualitative data-collection methods appropriate for a given public health context.

Planning and Management to Promote Health
- Assess population needs, assets, and capacities that affect communities' health.
- Apply awareness of cultural values and practices to the design or implementation of public health policies or programs.

REFERENCES

1. Corbin JM, Strauss AL. *Basics of Qualitative Research: Techniques and Procedures for Developing Grounded Theory.* 4th ed. Washington, DC: Sage Publishing; 2015. Accessed January 22, 2019. https://us.sagepub.com/en-us/nam/basics-of-qualitative-research/book235578

2. Willis K, Green J, Daly J, et al. Perils and possibilities: achieving best evidence from focus groups in public health research. *Aust N Z J Public Health.* 2009;33(2):131–136. doi:10.1111/j.1753-6405.2009.00358.x

3. Chan L, Taber J, Oh A, et.al. "Keep it realistic": reactions to and recommendations for physical activity promotion messaged from focus groups of women. *Am J Health Promot.* 2019;33(6):903–911. doi:10.1177/0890117119826870

4. Brown SA, Perkison WB, Garcia AA, et al. The Starr County border health initiative: focus groups on diabetes prevention in Mexican Americans. *Diabetes Educ.* 2018;44(3):293–306. doi:10.1177/0145721718770143

5. Camenga DR, Cavallo DA, Kong G, et.al. Adolescents' and young adults' perception of electronic cigarettes for smoking cessation: a focus group study. *Nicotine Tob Res.* 2015;17(10):1235–1241. doi:10.1093/ntr/ntv020

6. Cohen AJ, Oatmen KE, Heisler M, et.al. Facilitators and barriers to supplemental nutritional assistance program incentive use: findings from a clinic intervention for low-income patients. *Am J Prev Med.* 2019;56(4):571–579. doi:10.1016/j.amepre.2018.11.010

7. Griffith DM, Brinkley-Rubinstein L, Bruce MA, et al. The interdependence of African American men's definitions of manhood and health. *Fam Community Health.* 2015;38(4):284–296. doi:10.1097/FCH.0000000000000079

8. Krueger R, Casey M. *Focus Groups: A Practical Guide for Applied Research.* 5th ed. Thousand Oaks, CA: Sage; 2015.

9. Stewart D, Shamdasani P, Rook D. Conducting the focus group. In: Stewart D, Shamdasani P, Rook D, eds. *Focus Groups: Theory and Practice.* 2nd ed. Thousand Oaks, CA: Sage; 2007:89–107.

10. Krippendorff K. *Content Analysis: An Introduction to Its Methodlogy.* 4th ed. Thousand Oaks, CA: Sage; 2019.

11. Israel BA, Schulz AJ, Parker EA, Becker AB. Review of community based research: assessing partnership approaches to improve public health. *Annu Rev Public Health.* 1998;19(1):173–202. doi:10.1146/annurev.publhealth.19.1.173

12. Wang C, Burris MA. Photovoice: concept, methodology, and use for participatory needs assessment. *Health Educ Behav.* 1997;24(3):369–387. doi:10.1177/109019819702400309

13. Spencer RA, McIsaac J-LD, Stewart M, et al. Food in focus: youth exploring food in schools using photovoice. *J Nutr Educ Behav.* 2019;51(8):1011–1019. doi:10.1016/j.jneb.2019.05.599

14. Baig AA, Stutz MR, Fernandez Piñeros P, et al. Using photovoice to promote diabetes self-management in Latino patients. *Transl Behav Med.*2019;9(6):1151–1156. doi:10.1093/tbm/ibz082

15. Cho S, Kim MA, Kwon SIL. Using the photovoice method to understand experiences of people with physical disabilities working in social enterprises. *Disabil Health J*. 2019;12(4):685–693. doi:10.1016/j. dhjo.2019.03.011

16. Eyler AA, Valko C, Serrano N. Perspectives on high school "pay to play" sports fee policies: a qualitative study. *Transl J Am Coll Sports Med*. 2018;3(19):152–157.

17. Hipp JA, Eyler AA. Open streets initiatives: measuring success toolkit. January 2014. Accessed November 8, 2019. https://activelivingresearch.org/open-streets-initiatives-measuring-success-toolkit

ADDITIONAL READINGS AND RESOURCES

Ciolan L, Manasia L. Reframing photovoice to boost its potential for learning research. *Int J Qual Methods*. 2017;16:1–15. doi:10.1177/1609406917702909

Grieb SD, Eder M, Smith KC, et al. Qualitative research and community-based participatory research: considerations for effective dissemination in the peer-reviewed literature. *Prog Community Health Partnersh*. 2015;9(2):275–282. doi:10.1353/cpr.2015.0041

Rabinowitz P. Windshield and walking surveys. Community Tool Box. Center for Community Health and Development, University of Kansas. 2020. Accessed September 6, 2020. https://ctb.ku.edu/en/table-of-contents/assessment/assessing-community-needs-and-resources/windshield-walking-surveys/main

Zhu X, Weigel P, Baloh J, et al. Mobilising cross-sector collaborations to improve population health in US rural communities: a qualitative study. *BMC Open*. 2019;9(11):e030983. doi:10.1136/bmjopen-2019-030983

Qualitative Data Analysis

Stories are just data with a soul.
—Brené Brown, PhD, MSW

INTRODUCTION

Qualitative data offers a source for deep understanding of behaviors, actions, thoughts, and experiences. Human nature makes each qualitative study unique. It is the distinctive qualities of the participants, researchers, and settings that bring nuance to qualitative data analysis. Although the results are less generalizable than those produced from experimental studies, qualitative findings play an important role in building evidence for public health programs, policies, and interventions.

There is no universally applicable method to use to analyze qualitative data. However, the variety of approaches and analytic strategies used in qualitative data analysis all have a common purpose: data reduction. Qualitative research produces large amounts of detailed data. A 1-hour interview may result in 15 to 20 pages of transcribed text. If a researcher conducts 15 interviews, that will yield 300 pages of information. Imagine disseminating 300 pages of text to your target audience. It would not be well received! It is up to the researcher to reduce data in order to reveal a more concise understanding, explanation, and interpretation of the people and settings being studied. The goals of qualitative data analysis are to efficiently and effectively create a summary that represents the whole data.

The process for analyzing qualitative data can be inductive, deductive, or a combination of the two. **Inductive analysis** starts with the data and works up to theoretical patterns and themes. This inductive approach allows a framework to emerge from the data itself. A **deductive approach** begins with some preconceived theory base or hypothesis, and the patterns and themes are used to show support for (or lack of) the preconceptions. In deduction, the research question guides how data are grouped and compared. Sometimes analysis includes both processes. Corbin and Strauss (2015) describe the grounded theory approach as both inductive and deductive. They suggest this is due to the researcher always having some form of preconceived thoughts as "no researcher enters the research process with a completely blank mind."[1] Selection of the most appropriate process to use for qualitative analysis should occur when developing the overall research goals.

Qualitative data analysis can be complex, challenging, and even intimidating to the novice researcher. The process relies oncritical thinking skills rather than a standard test for statistical significance. Also adding to the complexity is the fact that qualitative data analysis is a nonlinear process. It is often depicted as a circular, spiral, or bidirectional process (Figure 13.1). The distinction between the phases of qualitative data collection and analysis is blurred because of the back-and-forth nature of the process. Initial analysis may reveal the need for more data in order to answer the research question, thus requiring revisiting the data-collection phase. This can occur several times throughout the study.

Quantitative researchers may be especially apprehensive about conducting qualitative data analysis. The lack of precision and concrete objectivity that are inherent in qualitative analysis are cause for concern for some quantitative methodologists. However, together quantitative and qualitative methods contribute to the body of evidence for improving complex public health issues. Public health students need training and skills in both analytical methodologies. Even if a public health biostatistician or epidemiologist may never conduct qualitative data analysis, knowing how the conclusions are determined and being able to assess the quality of qualitative studies contribute to a comprehensive methodological skill set.

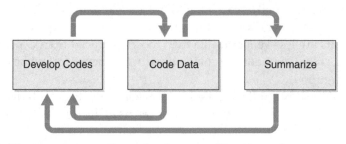

FIGURE 13.1 **The process of analyzing qualitative data**

PREPARING DATA FOR QUALITATIVE ANALYSIS

Audio/video recording is commonly used to capture data in qualitative research. To prepare the data for analysis, the recordings need to be transcribed or written into text form. Transcription should capture more than just audible talk. "How" things are said (e.g., emphasis, tone, pauses) provide important contextual details. Consider the following example taken from a study on interactions between diabetes educators and overweight, prediabetic young adults. The following transcription only includes audible talk as written words.

> DE1: According to your food records, yes. Yes you could improve the intake, eat more vegetables you know.
> PT1: No way. I hate vegetables unless they are deep fried or slathered in ranch dressing. Ha ha.

To make the data more comprehensive, details on pauses, emphasis, and body language are added to the same transcription example.

> DE1: (…) Um, according to your food records (…) yes. Yes you could improve the intake, (…) Eat more vegetables (…) you know?
> PT1: NO (…) WAY! (Hands up and palms out) (…) Uh I HATE vegetables unless they are deep-fried or slathered in ranch dressing. (Arms crossed against body)

With the details added, the transcription reflects both what is said and how it is said. It is up to the researcher to decide on the level of transcript detail needed for appropriate data analysis. In addition to details, it is necessary to determine what counts as data. For example, will small talk before the interview begins be considered data? Will side conversations unrelated to the study topic be considered data? Also, how will data be de-identified? Will names of people and places be omitted? It is helpful to keep all data intact in an original document, and then, after decisions are made about what will be analyzed, to create an edited transcript, which reflects only the data to be used for analysis.

Some researchers or students in qualitative training may opt to transcribe files themselves. However, precise transcribing is a skill that can be time-consuming. Depending on the level of skill, transcribing the recording can take up to four times the length of the actual audio file. If an interview lasts an hour, it may take 4 hours to accurately transcribe the conversation. Advancements in audio-file technology (e.g., the ability to listen at slow speeds or easily stop and start) can make the transcribing process more manageable. Another option is to use software programs specifically designed for transcription. There are several from which to choose, ranging in price and capacity. Advancements in word-recognition technology have improved these programs, but the transcripts should be double-checked for accuracy. A third option is to use a professional transcription service. This is likely the most convenient, but also the most costly option. Pricing structures for transcription vary. Transcriptionists can charge fees per audio minute or hour, per line of text produced, per typed page, or per hour of work time. This method is efficient, as audio or video files can be sent to the transcriptionist online, and they will return a text file in the desired format. It is best to get recommendations for quality transcription services from colleagues or resources in a university research office.

Whichever methods of transcription you choose, reliability checks are important to ensure accurate data capture. Randomly choose segments of the audio or video files and read over the corresponding transcript to identify the accuracy between the spoken words and the written text. Even though there is some level of interpretation needed to transform spoken words into text, there should be few discrepancies between the two formats. Document strategies for ensuring reliability in methodological notes so this information can be added to the research report.

Once transcription is completed, the next step in preparing data for qualitative analysis is to gather all the information together. Compile transcripts, process notes, observational data, and methods reports. If the research is a team effort, all members should review the aggregated data. Develop strategies for data access and storage. Even details on how to name files are important to determine prior to analysis. Finally, revisit study aims and research questions to provide focus for the next steps.

SUMMARY OF QUALITATIVE DATA ANALYSIS

1. Prepare data.
   - Transcribe if applicable.
   - Compile project documents.
   - Share with research team members.
   - Review study aims and research questions.
2. Code data.
   - Read through all transcripts.
   - Create the initial code list.
   - Practice coding, revise list (may be done multiple times).
   - Generate code book with definitions and examples.
   - Code data, using constant comparison coding if needed.
   - Conduct reliability checks of more than one coder and determine consensus.
3. Review data by codes.
   - Develop themes.
   - Identify relationships among codes or categories.
   - Determine whether important concepts are missing.
   - Conduct second-level coding if appropriate.
4. Summarize data.
   - Create summary table.
   - Develop an outline of the way you will present the findings.
   - Use quotes to represent themes and concepts if relevant.
   - Connect findings to their relevance for research and practice.
   - Compare and contrast results with other studies (both qualitative and quantitative).

CODING QUALITATIVE DATA

Data reduction begins with organizing text into meaningful categories using a process called **coding**. Coding adds structure to analysis by providing labels to words, phrases, and sentences. Adu (2013) defines coding as a systematic and subjective, transparent process of reducing data to meaningful and credible concepts that adequately represent the data and address the research problem, purpose, or question.[2] The researcher creates a list of codes based on inductive or deductive processes, and assigns the codes to parts of the text. This helps group similar text together.

Text from interviews with women at high risk for breast cancer about their preventative behaviors might be categorized using codes such as "diet," "physical activity," "mental health," and so on. In this very simplified example, codes could be applied as shown in Exhibit 13.1. In this example, the lines are numbered and text within those lines is assigned a corresponding code. Note that the text "I still drink my nightly glass of red wine though (laughs)." could be coded as part of the subsequent mental health quote in addition to being coded as diet. Text can be assigned more than one code in qualitative analysis.

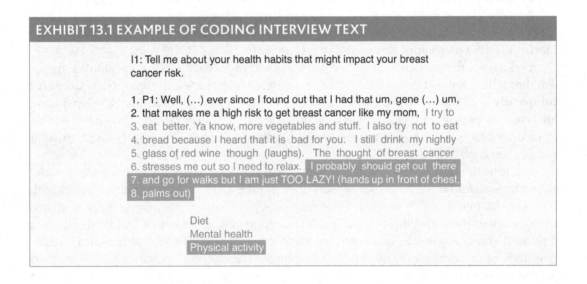

EXHIBIT 13.1 EXAMPLE OF CODING INTERVIEW TEXT

I1: Tell me about your health habits that might impact your breast cancer risk.

1. P1: Well, (…) ever since I found out that I had that um, gene (…) um,
2. that makes me a high risk to get breast cancer like my mom, I try to
3. eat better. Ya know, more vegetables and stuff. I also try not to eat
4. bread because I heard that it is bad for you. I still drink my nightly
5. glass of red wine though (laughs). The thought of breast cancer
6. stresses me out so I need to relax. I probably should get out there
7. and go for walks but I am just TOO LAZY! (hands up in front of chest,
8. palms out)

Diet
Mental health
Physical activity

Description-based coding describes the content of the data such as specific actions, behaviors, or experiences of participants. If a research study aims to explore public safety issues in a community park, description-based coding might reveal behaviors residents use to protect themselves such as walking in groups, carrying mace, staying on lighted paths, and so on. **Interpretation-based coding** goes a little deeper to explore and explain specific actions, behaviors, or experiences of participants. Interpretation-based coding might reveal themes or concepts on why residents choose specific strategies to protect themselves. Many studies use a combination of description and interpretation for comprehensive insight into the topic of study.

Deciding how to code data is almost as complex as the task itself, as there are many different typologies of coding presented in the qualitative data-analysis literature. Many qualitative public health studies start with either open coding or focused coding. **Open coding** is the basis of grounded theory. According to Corbin and Strauss, open coding is defined as breaking apart and delineating concepts to stand for interpreted meaning of raw data.[1] The research is "open" to find whatever is present in the data, rather than starting with a preconceived list of codes. Using the open-coding strategy, the researcher reads over the data multiple times to look for emergent concepts and themes. Comparisons and contrasts are made among these initial ideas, which helps to create more details to clarify and enrich the analysis. Focused coding is more deductive. In **focused coding**, codes are created a priori, or preceding the initial concept and theory development. Suppose you are conducting interviews with young adults seeking treatment for sexually transmitted diseases in order to inform intervention strategies. From the literature, you know which concepts in behavior change models are especially relevant to safe-sex practices. You may start with a list of theoretically based codes such as beliefs, attitudes, social norms, and perceived control. With focused coding, these codes provide the basis of text categorization. Once codes are developed, the researcher may choose to do **axial coding**, in which the data are assembled in new ways by combining codes or making connections across categories. Axial coding is a second-level analysis, like a "code of codes." For example, codes of barriers to mammography screening (e.g., knowledge about risk, lack of insurance coverage, lack of access, etc.) may be grouped together in axial codes such as "personally modifiable" or "systems modifiable." Piecing together data supports thematic development.

Coding is a fluid process. Whether you use open or focused coding, constant comparison throughout the coding process enhances comprehensiveness and consistency. **Constant comparative analysis** is applied when new codes or ways to categorize data develop during analysis. The previously coded data is then re-analyzed to incorporate the new codes. As this re-analysis process continues, the need for modifications eventually diminishes and constant comparison is no longer needed.

Public health researchers commonly use several coding strategies within the same analysis, each one contributing to unique aspects of the overall analysis and thematic development. For example, in a study on neighborhood factors of physical activity among Black residents living in low-income neighborhoods, Child et al. reports using both open and axial coding to develop themes.[3] Harte et al. used both open and focused coding to analyze data in a qualitative study of mealtimes in early childhood settings.[4] The decision on which coding method (or combination of methods) to use should be informed by your overall research goals and best practices related to your topic and population.

To keep the process organized and transparent and guide data analysis, many qualitative researchers create codebooks to guide data analysis (Table 13.1). **Codebooks** document all codes and definitions, and sometimes offer examples of text in which the codes are applicable. See Exhibit 13.2 for a codebook example from a study on advocates' use of research to inform efforts of policy change. A well-developed codebook is especially useful for projects for which more than one person will be coding data, as it may serve as a training tool for research team members, and can be used to foster inter-rater reliability.

TABLE 13.1 EXAMPLE OF A QUALITATIVE ANALYSIS CODEBOOK		
#	Title	Definition
1	Background	General background not including title and agency, which will be put into a separate spreadsheet
1.1	Role in advocacy	Include both role of the agency as a whole or a description of the individual's role

(continued)

TABLE 13.1 EXAMPLE OF A QUALITATIVE ANALYSIS CODEBOOK (*continued*)

#	Title	Definition
1.2	Length of time working in advocacy	Include description of length of time in years or history of participant's advocacy role
1.3	Unique role	Code here if cancer survivor or other unique reason that the person is in the advocacy role
2	Success	Include general comments here (e.g. luck, hard to say, etc.)
2.1	Collaboration/ relationships/ partnerships	Code this if describing relations with policy makers, volunteers, liaisons, other organizations who contribute to successful advocacy
2.2	Communication factors	Code if describing successful ways of communicating * will also be discussed in #3
2.3	Knowledge	Code if describing issue history, facts, good arguments, being well-informed
2.4	Good planning, persistence	Code if describing how advocacy was planned, staying focused on issue, etc.
2.5	Other factors	Code if describing factors about the organization, government, or specific things mentioned that contribute to success
2.6	Representative quote	This is a phrase of statement exemplifying success
3	Learning what works	General comments on what works
3.1	General experience	Time, other jobs
3.2	Trial and error	Code if specific mention of trial and error
3.3	On-the-job training or workshops	Describes specific courses, webinars, or trainings on advocacy NOT part of formal education
3.4	Formal education	Degree, internships

(continued)

TABLE 13.1 EXAMPLE OF A QUALITATIVE ANALYSIS CODEBOOK (*continued*)

#	Title	Definition
3.5	Relationships	With policy makers, mentors, coworkers
3.6	Self-education	Reading, self-taught, information from internet
3.7	Representative quote	A phrase or statement exemplifying learning what works
4	Using research	General comments of research
4.1	Individual research	Does own research as part of job and interprets topics and literature
4.2	Organizational research	Organization that individual works for conducts research
4.3	Other organization's or professional research	Code if mention of using research conducted by other organizations, including universities; also include if mention of specialty such as epidemiologist, etc.
4.4	Description of source of research	Credible, realistic, or other descriptors
4.5	Representative quote	A phrase or statement exemplifying use of research
5	Barriers	Describes factors which make communicating and advocacy challenging
5.1	Political will	Characteristics associated with the policy maker such as party affiliation, re-election concerns, ideology, perception of constituent concern, or support
5.2	Political climate	Describes the state or locality (e.g., personal responsibility, conservative, anti-tax, etc.), bad timing
5.3	Opposition	Organization or individual
5.4	Financial barriers	Code for organizational or general budget/funding concerns
5.5	Lack of relationships	Code for no access to policy makers or other resources that would help success

(*continued*)

TABLE 13.1 EXAMPLE OF A QUALITATIVE ANALYSIS CODEBOOK (*continued*)

#	Title	Definition
5.6	Lack of information, preparation, communication	Code used to mention not enough info is available, accessible, or offers an effective message
5.7	Representative quote	A phrase or statement exemplifying learning what works
6	Making research more useful	Describes overall factors for making research better suited for usability
6.1	Understandable	Offers better clarity and language in research information
6.2	Quality	Important, credible
6.3	Stories/personal	Describes adding stories to communication
6.4	Access	Updated, timely, easily accessible
6.5	Data	Includes state or local data, statistics
6.6	Consider fiscal impact	Include information about how this impacts budget or cost
6.7	Representative quote	A phrase or statement exemplifying making research more useful

EXHIBIT 13.2 CODEBOOK EXAMPLE

The following example is an excerpt from a codebook using focused coding.

Code Number	Opposition	Definition	Example of Relevant Text
7.0	Opposition to health curriculum changes	Opposition to modifying the existing health education curriculum in the district	*"There are a lot of people around here who get really upset when schools do things that don't match personal beliefs."*

(continued)

EXHIBIT 13.2 CODEBOOK EXAMPLE *(continued)*

Code Number	Opposition	Definition	Example of Relevant Text
7.1	Opposing groups	Specific groups opposing the sports participation fees	*"Parents, especially those trying to protect their kids from the big, bad world, are especially vocal about their opposition."*
7.2	Addressing opposition	How opposition to the curriculum changes are addressed	*"School admin holds lots of public meetings to ease their minds and show them that we are using evidence-based ways to educate kids."*
7.2.1	Addressing opposing parents	How the district/school addressed opposing parents	*"We now have an online feedback system. Kind of like a blog, where parents can voice their concerns and make recommendations."*
7.2.2	Addressing opposing school personnel	How the district/school addressed opposing personnel	*"We solicit teacher feedback well before we make any decisions."*

THE TEAM APPROACH IN QUALITATIVE DATA ANALYSIS

There are several benefits to having a research team when analyzing qualitative data. Having multiple coders provides multiple perspectives. This approach widens the lens of an individual researcher and enhances reflexivity in the qualitative process. Qualitative data analysis is a complex, time-consuming process. Multiple coders can reduce individual workloads. With proper training for consistency across coders, the team can divide and conquer the data. Some helpful steps include the following:

- Read overall data individually to draft a list of main codes.
- Meet to discuss all coding ideas, and compile the first iteration of the code list.

- Code a small sample of data (e.g., transcripts from one interview) together.
- Refine code list.
- Code another small sample of data independently.
- Review consistency and reach consensus on any discrepancies.
- Develop codebook.
- Divide coding assignments.
- Establish the amount of data to be coded by two people for reliable documentation.

There are several different ways to implement the coding process. Researchers have options such as manual approaches, using word-processing or database programs, or utilizing computer programs specifically designed to analyze qualitative data. Each has advantages and disadvantages, and factors, such as amount of data, researcher experience, budget, and timeline, are issues to consider when selecting the method of qualitative data analysis.

Manual Approaches

Qualitative researchers can opt to code the data "by hand." This method works best for smaller amounts of data, or data from a single source (i.e., all data from interviews). The manual approach begins with a printout of transcripts, whereby the researcher can use a variety of ways to code and sort the data. Some researchers cut the transcripts into pieces of data corresponding to the codes. The pieces are then grouped together visually to aid in concept and theme development. Wallboards are especially useful for this process. Digital photos can also be used to capture visual images of the sorting. Other researchers opt to use colors to match code with corresponding text. Manual approaches are sometimes recommended for beginning researchers so they can experience and understand the full extent of the coding process. The hands-on approach of this method enhances the interaction between researcher and data, but requires good organizational skills.

Word-Processing/Database Approaches

Researchers can opt to use word-processing programs (e.g., Microsoft Word) or database programs (Excel) to facilitate qualitative data coding. One way to do this in Word is to highlight relevant text and insert a comment bubble containing the corresponding code (Exhibit 13.3A). Another option is to highlight the text and insert the code name or number in parentheses after the applicable word, phrase, sentence(s) within the document (Exhibit 13.3B). To retrieve all text within a certain code, the "find" tool will show all places in the document where that code was placed. Some researchers opt to use databases to store and organize coded text. This involves cutting the text to be coded and pasting it into a spreadsheet. The text can be pasted into separate code pages to enable the researcher to see all text within each code. Word-processing and database approaches are good options for researchers who are uncomfortable using the full manual approach. Also, computer files are more easily shared with research team members than cut or colored-coded text. However, computer-based coding methods still take time, consistency, and organizational skills.

EXHIBIT 13.3 EXAMPLE OF USING IN-TEXT COMMENTS OR HIGHLIGHTS TO CODE

I1: Tell me about your health habits that might impact your breast cancer risk.

A.

1. P1: Well, (. . .) ever since I found out that I had that um, gene (. . .) um,
2. that makes me a high risk to get breast cancer like my mom, I try to
3. eat better. Ya know, more vegetables and stuff. I also try not to eat
4. bread because I heard that it is bad for you. I still drink my nightly
5. glass of red wine though (laughs). The thought of breast cancer
6. stresses me out so I need to relax. I probably should get out there
7. and go for walks but I am just TOO LAZY! (hands up in front of chest,
8. palms out)

    3. Diet
    2. Mental health
    3. Physical Activity

B.

1. P1: Well, (. . .) ever since I found out that I had that um, gene (. . .) um,
2. that makes me a high risk to get breast cancer like my mom, I try to
3. eat better. Ya know, more vegetables and stuff. I also try not to eat
4. bread because I heard that it is bad for you. I still drink my nightly
5. glass of red wine though, (laughs). The thought of breast cancer
6. stresses me out so I need to relax. I probably should get out there
7. and go for walks but I am just TOO LAZY! (hands up in front of chest,
8. palms out)

    1
    1 and 2
    2
    3

Qualitative-Analysis Software

Computer programs specifically designed for qualitative analysis have evolved over the past few decades. Once limited in function and availability, qualitative researchers now use these programs widely. Several different programs exist, each with slightly different functions, but similar processes. Transcripts or other data files are imported into the program, along with the coding scheme. Similar to using a word-processing program, the coder highlights the relevant text and assigns that section the corresponding code. All text under each code can be easily grouped together, with the source of each code noted. One benefit is the ease in which large amounts of qualitative data can be stored and organized. Multiple people can have access to the files, making these programs a good choice for larger research teams. In spite of the advantages, these programs can be costly and require user training.

Some researchers may opt to use a combination of these methods to code data. In a large qualitative study of administrative evidence-based practices in state health departments, Eyler et al. used both software and manual methods to code data. Researchers first coded all text using NVivo, a qualitative software analysis program. All text that was initially coded in the software program under the code "equity" was separated and printed. The printed text was then hand coded to identify ways in which equity was prioritized and operationalized within state health departments.[5] Using hybrid methods, such as the one used in this example, can compensate for advantages and disadvantages of singular methods.

Whichever coding method is used, memos or side notes about the process provide useful documentation for other steps in the qualitative research process. Memos may be justifications for the ways in which codes were developed, omitted, merged, or changed. They can also include operational notes such as how the research team determined consensus in coding or reliability strategies. Researchers should also note initial thoughts and reflections about themes and concepts while coding. Anyone involved in data analysis should keep memos and notes for sharing with the research team.

REVIEWING AND SUMMARIZING QUALITATIVE DATA

One of the highlights of qualitative research is discovering patterns in the data. The perseverance required to go through iterations of coding and recoding results in recognizing the emergent meanings and insights the data offers. Lofland et al. suggest six different types of patterns to seek in coded qualitative data.[6] Suppose you conducted interviews with older adults about fall prevention. Some questions to guide exploration of these types of patterns might include the following:

> Frequencies: How often do older adults practice home/neighborhood fall-prevention strategies?
> Magnitudes: What is the extent of the risk present in their homes or neighborhoods?
> Structures: What are the different types of risks?
> Processes: How do certain risks coincide with phases of aging or comorbidities of the population?
> Causes: What do older adults perceive as the causes of falling?
> Consequences: How does falling impact the lives of older adults? What would fall prevention strategies do to change these consequences?

Another pattern to look for in qualitative data is the absence of certain factors. What was *not* said can be informative, too. In the example study on fall prevention, maybe only individuals in certain neighborhoods talked about poor sidewalk conditions. This type of information is useful for making recommendations to target program, intervention, or policies strategies. Any type of pattern may emerge in data from individuals and across participants or participant groups. Noting similarities and differences within and across individuals and groups is useful for developing summaries and conclusions.

One factor confusing to the novice qualitative researcher (and even some with more advanced research skills) is quantification of qualitative data. Counting or quantifying the number of times a code is present in the data or how many individuals or groups mentioned the code or concept is typically not a qualitative-analysis strategy, yet this information is often requested by reviewers or stakeholders. Consider this simplistic example. In a study on weight-loss strategies of low-income, Hispanic women who are obese, one participant stated:

> "I hate exercise! Exercise, exercise, exercise. Blah, blah, blah. That is all I hear from my doctor. You need to exercise more. My mom is telling me I should walk for exercise. She is always telling me how exercise will help me lose weight."

In this example, the word "exercise" was used seven times. Is knowing that the word was used seven times meaningful? No. The word should be noted in the context of the whole statement. If one woman just said "I hate exercise" and another goes into in-depth explanation of her exercise history, would these two "counts" be considered equal? No. Interpretation and context are more applicable than quantification in most qualitative data analysis. Quantifying qualitative data may result in inaccurate conclusions. However, in limited instances, such as analyzing open-ended question responses, quantification may be relevant.

The goal of coding is data reduction. Summaries condense a large amount of data into patterns, concepts, and themes easily that are understandable to others not involved in the research project. An effective way to visualize patterns and themes is to develop a table. See Table 13.2 for a template of what might be included in a summary table. Tables can include patterns, summary notes, and text or quotes that exemplify the pattern. The condensed data organized into a table is a good resource for developing final summaries and conclusions.

Use the table information to create an outline for the summary narrative. The outline helps plan a logical flow of results. Information from memos and notes can also be added as details to expand the outline. Quotes are also an effective addition to the summary. Each main outline section can be represented by relevant, direct quotes from the data. Quotes are effective in humanizing the research results, and are a way to demonstrate the value of participant contribution in the qualitative research process. Highlighting quotes is a great way to emphasize themes in presentations and other dissemination methods. For peer-reviewed publications, journal requirements may impact how quotes are displayed. Some prefer the quotes to be presented in text, others recommend putting the representative quotes in a corresponding table. Using a table also helps keep within word limits as required by some public health journals. Match the style of quote presentation with the dissemination type and target audience.

TABLE 13.2 TEMPLATE FOR A QUALITATIVE DATA-SUMMARY TABLE

Concept or Theme	Supporting Evidence From Data	Relationship With Other Concepts or Themes	Example Quote
1.			
2.			
3.			

The expanded outline should evolve into a report, which summarizes and represents the larger body of data. Some reports also include information on how results may relate to other studies (both qualitative and quantitative) on similar topics. The importance of methodological details or research limitations will vary by dissemination target. Tailor the reports to the target audience, as peer-reviewed literature differs from white papers and evaluation reports. Details on best practices for dissemination and visualization of results are presented in Chapter 14, Summarizing and Visualizing Data, and in Chapter 15, Disseminating Research Results.

Good qualitative data analysis will provide answers to the following questions:

- What patterns and themes occur?
- What are deviations from the patterns and themes?
- What is missing from patterns and themes?
- What is the relationship among the patterns and themes?
- What compelling stories emerge?
- Is more data collection needed?
- How do findings compare to other studies?

CHAPTER DISCUSSION QUESTIONS

1. How might developing different codes affect the way themes are developed?
2. Discuss the pros and cons of manual transcription, word-processing/database, and qualitative-analysis software.
3. How could the way things are said (in addition to *what* is said) be included in qualitative analysis? Describe an example of a demographic group or public health topic for which this might be particularly important.
4. What strategies could you implement to ensure reliable and rigorous qualitative data analysis?

RESEARCH PROJECT CHECK-IN

Reduce, Reuse, Recycle

Data reduction is the ultimate goal of qualitative analysis, but it's not as simple as it sounds. Qualitative research produces large amounts of data, and chances are there will be some back and forth between data collection and analysis. Choose which approach you will use to analyze your data before starting to reduce the data by coding and thematic development. Keep in mind that the researcher is a big part of interpretation in qualitative analysis. Use best practices for reducing bias and addressing reflexivity. Keep your eye out for key quotes representing themes. They are useful for dissemination.

PUBLIC HEALTH RESEARCH METHODS IN REAL LIFE

Pencil or Processor?

Korrie knew her boss had a background in anthropology and had conducted several ethnographical studies decades ago during her doctoral studies. Dr. Salomon's expertise came in handy when their division was asked to conduct a qualitative study of state public health practitioners working in breast and cervical cancer prevention (BCCP) programs. The aims of the study were to explore the need for technical assistance and assess ways to enhance resource sharing. Korrie also had qualitative research experience. In her previous job, she was the qualitative data analyst for a small research center. Together they planned a study in which they would interview BCCP project managers in every state. One thing they didn't discuss was analysis. Korrie assumed they would use qualitative software, yet Dr. Salomon assumed they would hand-code and analyze the data.

They used a list of all state BCCP program practitioners for recruitment. Most states had two practitioners, with a few of the larger states having up to five. They decided to randomly select and recruit two practitioners in the larger states for a total of 75 interviews, with representation from each state. They developed and tested the interview questions with the help of the BCCP program staff in their own state. Once revised and finalized, Korrie and her boss conducted telephone interviews. Over the course of 3 months, they completed data collection.

They digitally recorded the interviews and had the files professionally transcribed. Each interviewer also typed up their process notes and attached them to the corresponding transcriptions. Since each interview lasted about an hour, the result was nearly 750 pages of transcribed text to analyze. Korrie was getting ready to upload the files into the qualitative-software program, when Dr. Salomon realized they had conflicting thoughts on how the data should be analyzed. Dr. Salomon was not opposed to using software, she just was unaware of the benefits of computer coding and analysis over doing the work by hand. Their progress came to an abrupt stop until they could come to a consensus. Dr. Salomon had an idea. She would use her past experience in hand-coding and analyzing to come up with a list of reasons they should do it by hand. Korrie would create a list in favor of using the software.

When they came back together, Dr. Salomon was proud to present her list. Her first reason to support by-hand coding and analysis was the intimacy a researcher has with the data when they read, highlight, cut, and organize the pieces of data. Her second reason was that a large portion of the data could be displayed at one time on, for example, the walls of a room. A computer screen could only show so much. She also mentioned that this method was more accepted among qualitative researchers than computer-aided analysis.

Korrie was ready to present her list and give a demonstration of the software to Dr. Salomon. Reading, highlighting, and cutting could be done with the software, with the advantages of searching within text and easily compiling coded text. Korrie's second reason was practicality. She reminded Dr. Salomon that they had 750 pages to code and reduce into themes. Paper copies of this large amount of text would be unwieldy, not to mention less environmentally friendly than computer-aided qualitative analysis. She refuted Dr. Salomon's reason of hand-analysis being a more accepted method by producing a reference list of qualitative studies in top public health journals for which data were analyzed using software. Korrie also added that it is easy to share coded data in computer files. Their separate coding could easily be compared for reliability.

With careful consideration of each other's preference, Korrie and Dr. Salomon decided to use qualitative-analysis software. In the end, Dr. Salomon was happy with the process and the results.

Critical Thinking Questions

1. Do you agree with the analysis method selected in this example? Why or why not?
2. What other ways could Korrie have convinced Dr. Salomon of the merits of computer-aided qualitative analysis?
3. In this example, Korrie and Dr. Salomon had 750 pages of text to analyze. How much text would be manageable to analyze by hand?
4. Qualitative-analysis software is evolving, and new features are constantly being added. What technological aspects of computer software could make it more desirable than coding and analyzing by hand?
5. How might you learn about the benefits and disadvantages of qualitative software programs?

COUNCIL ON EDUCATION FOR PUBLIC HEALTH FOUNDATIONAL KNOWLEDGE AND COMPETENCIES

Foundational Knowledge

Profession and Science of Public Health

- Explain the critical importance of evidence in advancing public health knowledge.
- Explain the role of quantitative and qualitative methods and sciences in describing and assessing a population's health.

Evidence-Based Approaches to Public Health

- Select quantitative and qualitative data-collection methods appropriate for a given public health context.

Planning and Management to Promote Health

- Assess population needs, assets, and capacities that affect communities' health.
- Apply awareness of cultural values and practices to the design or implementation of public health policies or programs.

REFERENCES

1. Corbin JM, Strauss AL. *Basics of Qualitative Research: Techniques and Procedures for Developing Grounded Theory.* 4th ed. Washington, DC: Sage Publishing; 2015. Accessed January 22, 2019. https://us.sagepub.com/en-us/nam/basics-of-qualitative-research/book235578

2. Adu P. *A Step-by-Step Guide to Qualitative Data Coding. 1st ed.* New York, NY: Routledge; 2019. Accessed October 26, 2019. doi:10.4324/9781351044516

3. Child ST, Kaczynski AT, Fair ML, et al. 'We need a safe, walkable way to connect our sisters and brothers': a qualitative study of opportunities and challenges for neighborhood-based physical activity among residents of low-income African-American communities. *Ethn Health.* 2019;24(4): 353–364. doi:10.1080/13557858.2017.1351923

4. Harte S, Theobald M, Trost SG. Culture and community: observation of mealtime enactment in early childhood education and care settings. *Int J Behav Nutr Phys Act.* 2019;16: 69.doi:10.1186/s12966-019-0838-x

5. Eyler AA, Valko C, Ramadas R, et al. Administrative evidence-based practices in state chronic disease practitioners. *Am J Prev Med.* 2018;54(2):275–283. doi:10.1016/j.amepre.2017.09.006

6. Lofland J, Snow DA, Anderson L, et al. *Analyzing Social Settings: A Guide to Qualitative Observation and Analysis.* 4th ed. Belmont, CA; Wadsworth Publishers; 2005.

ADDITIONAL READINGS AND RESOURCES

Lofland J, Snow DA, Anderson L, et al. *Analyzing Social Settings: A Guide to Qualitative Observation and Analysis.* 4th ed. Belmont, CA; Wadsworth Publishing; 2005.

Osborg Ose S. Using excel and word to structure qualitative data. *J Appl Soc Sci.* 2016;10(2):147–162. doi:10.1177/1936724416664948

Otten JJ, Dodson EA, Fleischhacker S, et al. Getting research to the policy table: a qualitative study with public health researchers on engaging with policy makers. *Prev Chronic Dis.* 2015;12:14056. doi:10.5888/pcd12.140546

V

VISUALIZING, MESSAGING, AND DISSEMINATING RESULTS

The ultimate goal of public health research is to build evidence, but evidence does little good if no one knows about it. Preparing and sharing research results is critical, but public health professionals often lack skills in effective visualization, messaging, and dissemination. This section outlines some of the basic elements needed to improve this skill set. Chapter 14 describes the importance of visualizing data, and depicts options for graphics to use to represent data categories such as trends, surveys, and comparisons. Chapter 15 describes some ideas for developing messages from research results, and tailoring those messages for different groups. This chapter also provides a framework for dissemination, which can be used for planning the best ways to spread the word about your findings, and tracking the reach of your efforts.

Summarizing and Visualizing Data

In school we learn a lot about language and math. On the language side we learn how to put words together into sentences and stories. With math, we learn to make sense of numbers. But it's rare that these two sides are paired. No one tells us how to tell stories with numbers . . . this leaves us poorly prepared for an important task that is increasingly in demand.

—Cole Nussbaumer Knaflic
author, *Storytelling with Data*

LEARNING OBJECTIVES

After reading this chapter, the reader will be able to

- Understand the importance of data visualization.
- Choose the most relevant visualization method for research data.
- Describe best practices for presenting data.

INTRODUCTION

The research process does not end with the calculation of study results. In fact, the steps *after* analysis can have the most impact on public health. Effectively communicating research results is vital to building evidence and influencing public health policies and practice. As important as it is, this is often the most difficult phase for many public health researchers. Without a design background or other training in data presentation, summarizing data in visually appealing ways while also maintaining the true representation of results can be challenging. Think about times when you sat through presentations or read reports with really poor graphical representations of data. The way the data were presented was likely cluttered, unclear, and led to confusion about the results. As researchers, we often are really good at planning for, collecting, and analyzing data, but fall short when it comes to presentation.

Making data more understandable through visualization is not a new strategy. Forms of graphs and maps have been used throughout history, some dating back to ancient Egypt. Statistical graphics and thematic mapping evolved rapidly during the first half of the 19th century, and continues to develop today.[1] Recent technological advances have made it easier to accumulate better and more data in research, and there is an increasing need for skills to turn the data into useful information. In public health, learning how to develop tables and figures for an academic audience is important, but broader impact will come from other ways to present data. The evident need for these skills is changing public health education. The revised Council on Education for Public Health (CEPH) foundational competencies for all accredited public health schools and programs now include the requirement for training in "interpreting results of data analysis for public health research, policy, and practice."[6]

Effective data visualization drives the viewer through a process of understanding (Figure 14.1).[2] This process involves perceiving, interpreting, and comprehending the information presented. Perception results in basic knowledge of *what* is shown such as high or low numbers, large or small differences, and how data are connected. The next stage in the process of understanding is interpretation. When a person interprets data visualization, they assign meaning to the information, such as significance or uniqueness. The third step is comprehension. In this part of the process, the meaning is made personal. It is here a person relates the information to themself or their own setting. Comprehension also allows for an understanding of next steps or actions to be taken based on the data.

Human brains process information more easily when it is presented in charts or graphs as compared to more complex formats.[3] Visuals also help people remember concepts better

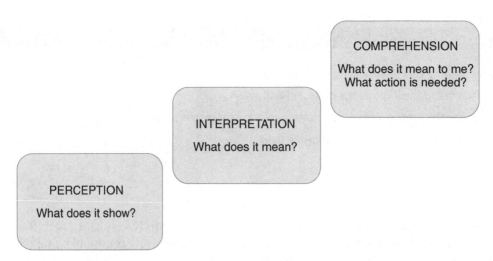

FIGURE 14.1 Data visualization facilitates progression through stages of understanding.

Source: Kirk, A. *Data Visualization*. Los Angeles: Sage; 2016. Accessed Nov 1, 2019. https://us.sagepub.com/sites/default/files/upm-binaries/75674_Kirk_Data_Visualisation.pdf[2]

than just words or numbers. With effective visualization, the target audience should be able to easily recall the significance of well-presented results. Graphical representation helps people quickly see and understand the importance of complex research results. In a world of ever-shortening attention spans, facilitating rapid comprehension of results is fundamental. Visualization also makes it easier to quickly discern patterns and trends within the data. Exhibit 14.1 shows a comparison of a data table and graphic representation of the same data. Although both the table and graph show the same information, a quick glance at the graph shows a relatively unchanged trend in flu vaccine uptake since 2010 to 2011. Presenting data in a way that people can understand quickly helps improve awareness of public health issues. Perhaps the awareness of the lack of improvement in vaccine use will stimulate new intervention strategies. Increased awareness and knowledge from effective visualization can influence support, prioritization, and public health decision-making.

Data visualization improves understanding of complex issues though clear and concise presentation. Visualization makes data more understandable and accessible to a broad audience. Effective data visualization facilitates an understanding of numerical information to all target audience groups, including researchers, stakeholders, policy makers, and community members. This is especially important when data can be used to impact decisions and policies to better serve the health needs of marginalized or vulnerable populations. Advocates and community members can become empowered with knowledge and evidence from well-designed visuals of data.

Organizations and government agencies are realizing the importance of data visualization for creating positive change. The Agency for Healthcare Research and Quality (AHRQ), a division of the U.S. Department of Health and Human Services, recently funded a program to

EXHIBIT 14.1 DATA (A) TABLE AND (B) GRAPHIC FOR ADULT FLU VACCINE UPTAKE 2010–2018

A

Season	Percentage of Adult Flu Vaccine Coverage
2010–2011	40.5
2011–2012	38.8
2012–2013	41.5
2013–2014	42.2
2014–2015	43.6
2015–2016	41.7
2016–2017	43.3
2017–2018	37.1

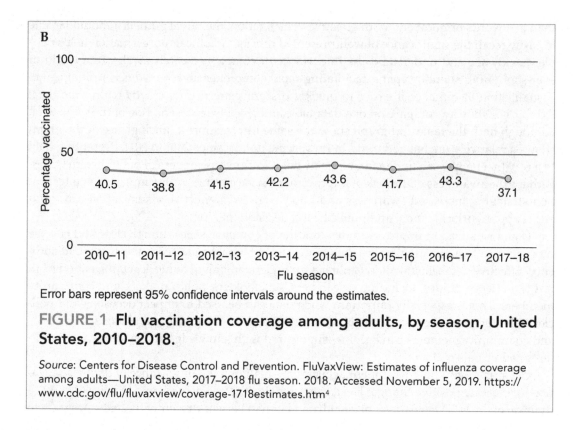

Error bars represent 95% confidence intervals around the estimates.

FIGURE 1 **Flu vaccination coverage among adults, by season, United States, 2010–2018.**

Source: Centers for Disease Control and Prevention. FluVaxView: Estimates of influenza coverage among adults—United States, 2017–2018 flu season. 2018. Accessed November 5, 2019. https://www.cdc.gov/flu/fluvaxview/coverage-1718estimates.htm[4]

facilitate creation of data visualization resources of community-level determinants of health (see www.ahrq.gov/sdoh-challenge/about.html). This program aims to improve health decision-making by increasing access to information through visual data resources. The U.S. Census provides many ways to visualize population data (www.census.gov/dataviz). The Centers for Disease Control and Prevention (CDC) has a long history of visualizing health data in disease surveillance and to show behavioral and outcome trends. The CDC is also improving the capacity for access to and ability to tailor data visualizations. CDC visuals are easily downloadable and can be used in intervention and advocacy efforts.

Diminishing resources and shifting priorities warrant strong and impactful messages from public health research. Consequently, data visualization skills are becoming increasingly important to many public health careers. Health departments, government agencies, nonprofit organizations, and corporations all have the need to reduce large amounts of complex data and turn it into meaningful and usable information. The demand for these skills is likely to grow as technological advances make it easier to collect and disseminate research data.

Technological advances have also improved the process of visualizing data. Programs such as Microsoft Excel make it easy for novice users to develop effective charts and graphics. The options for visualization are even greater for those with advanced Excel skills. Quantitative statistics programs, such as SPSS, SAS, and R, all have built-in graphic capabilities. The visuals created with these programs can easily be copied and pasted into documents, reports, or presentations. There are also software programs specifically made to develop graphics. Using programs such as Adobe InDesign or Illustrator may require training, but these software skills are helpful when complex public health data representation is needed.

DATA VISUALIZATION

Data visualizations are visual depictions of measured numbers or text through a combination of lines, shapes, points, or other symbols. This broad definition brings light to the multitude of ways data can be visualized. How do you choose the best way to present your data? Before selecting a bar chart over trend line, consider what you want the audience to know and how you want them to respond. Effective data visualization begins with identifying the intent or purpose of the visual. What research results do you want to emphasize? Each visual you develop should be based on a preconceived intent. As indicated in Figure 14.1, the last stage of the process of understanding is comprehension. In addition to your intent, also consider this: What is the takeaway message you hope for? What are the desired actions or next steps? Clarifying these issues will help guide your choice of data-visualization options.

There are many different ways to visualize the same data. Imagine how you could show the percentage of pregnant women in a community who intend to breastfeed compared to national data. You could make a table, a graph, or a chart, or use a picture. All of these choices would have the same goal of highlighting the lower rate in Anytown, United States, compared to national data. Which one is the best choice? The best format should offer a truthful representation of the data, be clear and concise, and be based on good design characteristics.

There are several main categories of data visualization. Each category is based on the intended purpose of the graphic. Although the list of suggestions offered within each category is not meant to be exhaustive, the overview can help inform your choice of visual.

Presenting Single Numbers

Sometimes research results boil down to one main finding for which a single number or one salient point is impactful. A simple representation of this number or point can be a powerful way to achieve the desired message. There are several options for visualizing a single number. Suppose you are reporting results from a study on the prevalence of people who live in food deserts. The most significant finding was that 80% of the 2,000 people surveyed reported living further than 10 miles from the nearest grocery store. Some options for depicting this single number are shown in Figure 14.2. Choice (A) shows a ratio (4/5), with font emphasis. This is an easy, yet impactful option. A single number can also be visualized using an appropriate icon. Choice (B) uses an icon of a grocery cart to represent data on food deserts. The figure 80% is shown through differences in shade of the grocery carts. A brief phrase is added to explain the graphic. Choice (C) is a pie chart. There are mixed reviews of effectiveness of pie charts as visuals in the graphic-design world, but here the chart quickly shows the vast difference in prevalence of living in a food desert and not living in a food desert. Pie charts work best for single numbers when the differences are large enough to easily understand just by looking at the proportional differences in the pie "slices." Choice (D) is a bar graph where the emphasis is on a single number. Manipulating color and font size make the number stand out in the graph.

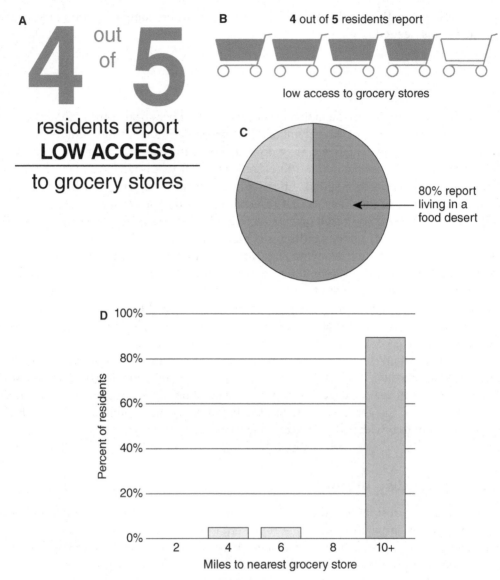

FIGURE 14.2 **Ways to present single numbers in an image.**

Comparisons

Public health research often involves comparisons, such as considering data from participants in a control group compared to an intervention group, or assessing similarities and differences across participant characteristics. Figure 14.3 shows different ways to visually represent simple data comparisons from a study on perception of cyberbullying among high school girls and boys. Results from this study indicate 67% of girls perceive cyberbullying as a significant problem in their school, compared with 30% of boys. Choice (A) is a side-by-side column graph. This works well for data with only two categories, such as in this cyberbullying example.

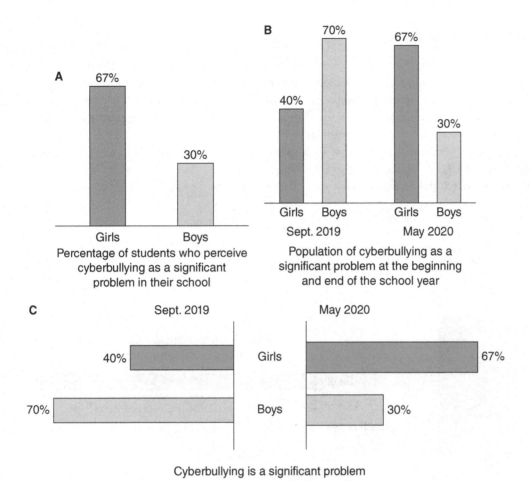

FIGURE 14.3 **Visualizing comparisons: (A) Side-by-side column graph, (B) slope graph, and (C) opposing bar graph**

Researchers may choose to add another variable (e.g., data from another school or district or national data), but too many groups can make the concepts more difficult to grasp quickly using side-by-side columns. Choice (B) is a slope graph. Slope graphs can show data from two or more variables, at one or more time points. From the cyberbullying study data, this slope graph depicts rates of girls and boys who think cyberbullying is a significant problem in their school at the beginning and end of the school year. This example shows the sharp increase in perception of girls, whereas the rate for boys remains relatively unchanged. Another option to show comparisons is the opposing bar graphs as in choice (C) in Figure 14.3. The bars can either be placed adjacent to one another or separated with the data label. In this example, each variable (only one—perception—is shown here) can be placed on a separate row, and data from two opposing groups are shown on either side. As with the other data visualization choices, there are many different ways to format and label graphs. Try a few different ways to come up with the best option.

Survey and Scale Results

Many public health research studies collect data through surveys. It can be challenging to turn the data from surveys into visuals, especially when you have many response options, missing data, and several subgroups of participants to represent. The goal of the visualization should be clear and concise communication of the survey results to inform understanding and action. Suppose you conduct a survey on community health assets. Figure 14.4 shows some options for depicting data from rating scales with sequential response options (e.g., excellent, good, poor). Choice (A) is the stacked bar graph. The variables are listed next to bars, which are subdivided to match the response categories. There should be adequate differentiation among

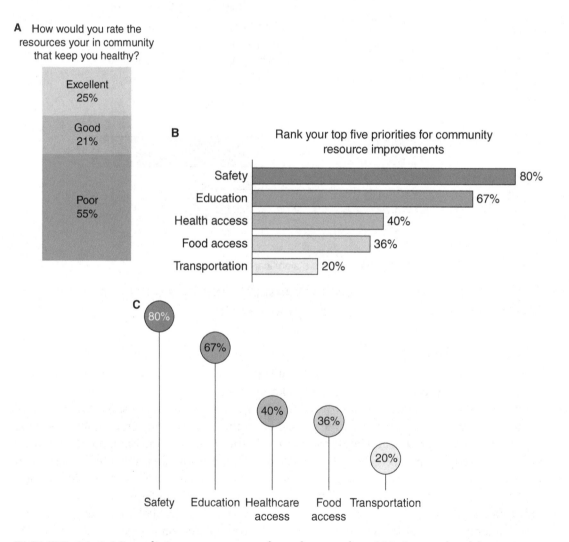

FIGURE 14.4 **Visualizing survey and scale results: (A) A stacked bar graph example, (B) a bar graph example, (C) example of a lollipop graph.**

categories using color or shading. Spaces or lines could also be used to separate categories. Choice (B) is one way to show ranking data. In the community health asset example, residents were asked to indicate their top areas of concern. They could respond with one or more answers. The responses are ranked from highest concern to lowest concern. You could choose to list all options, or reduce the number of categories displayed to those of most importance. Choice (C) is called a *lollipop graph*. This graph uses a line and a dot (when paired they look like a lollipop!) to show the same data as in Choice (B). Instead of bars, a marker highlights actual data values, which then are connected by a line to the variable category label.

Trends

Trends show the extent to which data changes over time. Data visualization of trends is similar to the types of graphics previously discussed, but can be slightly more complex due to the use of multiple time points. Let's say you are studying the impact of sugar-sweetened beverage taxes on purchases in intervention and comparison cities. You have monthly sugar-sweetened beverage sales data from both cities for 2 months before and 3 months after the tax was implemented. Figure 14.5 shows different ways to depict trends over time. Choice (A) is the line graph. Each line represents a city and dots indicate data points. The line helps the reader identify visual patterns. In this case, the city with the sugar-sweetened beverage tax had a decrease in sales for the 3 months following implementation, whereas sales in the comparison city changed very little during the same time period. Another way to show time trends is shown in B. The area graph is useful for data that can be pieced together to make up an entire unit. For the sugar-sweetened- beverage-tax example, suppose you have all beverage sales data for the same time period as in A. The area graph shows the changes in the different categories of beverages. Rather than data points and lines, the graph area uses solid colors or shading to depict the changes in different beverage categories. The choice of line or area graph will depend on the type of data and the type of story you want to tell.

Visualizing Qualitative Data

Data visualization is not only used for numbers. Qualitative research results can also be visually enhanced in several different ways. Word clouds (Figure 14.6) show the frequency of main words or phrases in text. Although this may seem like an option for qualitative research results, representation of quantitative results should be used with caution. As discussed in Chapter 13, Qualitative Data Analysis, merely counting words or phrases leaves out the importance of context of those words or phrases and misrepresents results. Other options for highlighting text results are shown in Figure 14.7. Let's use data from a public health study on worksite wellness. In an example study, you conducted interviews, focus groups, and observations to explore ways employees participate in healthy behaviors while at work. Emphasizing quotes or comments can be an effective way to break up text in written reports and represent data in presentations. Choice A shows a quote and a corresponding icon. Choice B is another option used to emphasize quotes by placing it in a callout box. Venn diagrams, as shown in C can visualize qualitative data. Venn diagrams are especially useful for comparing two groups. In the worksite example, you compared themes among men and women and found some similarities and differences. A Venn diagram could show the

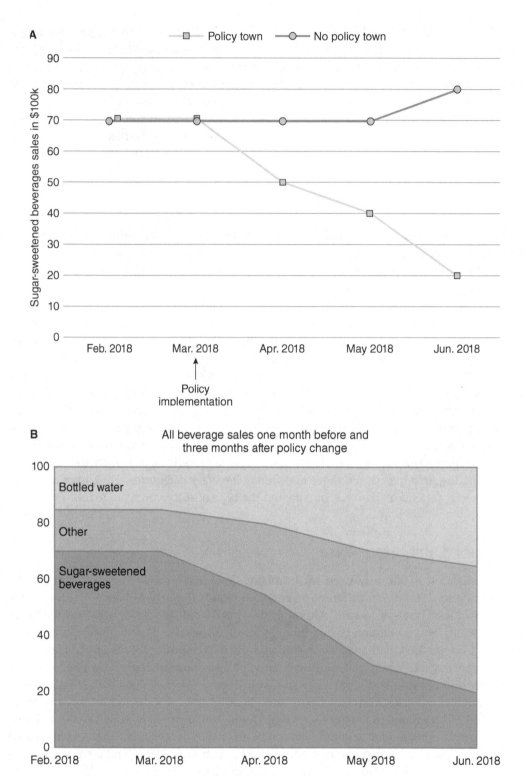

FIGURE 14.5 **Visualizing trends. (A) Example of a line graph and (B) example of an area graph.**

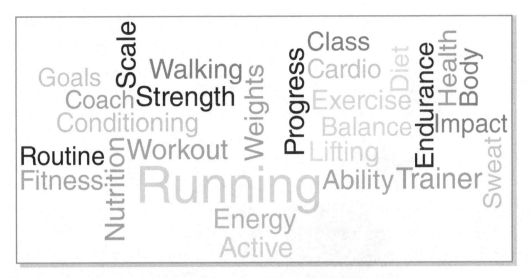

FIGURE 14.6 **Visualizing qualitative data: WordCloud**

similarities in the shared space, and the differences in themes in the separate circles. Choice D is a visual showing main themes and examples of how the themes were represented in the data. All of these qualitative data visualization options can enhance the impact of dissemination efforts by allowing the audience to quickly grasp the most salient results.

INFOGRAPHICS

Infographics (information graphics) are a form of data visualization that combines data with a narrative or story. Infographics can be effective in getting messages across to a broad audience. The visual stories provide an information overview to help viewers understand the concepts and quickly ascertain any patterns or trends. The CDC develops and provides infographics on a variety of public health topics as a way to get information to a wide-ranging audience. See Exhibit 14.2 for an example of an infographic on the changes in portion sizes over time. The CDC infographics can be downloaded, and used in interventions, campaigns, or advocacy efforts. Many other public health agencies also use these graphic messages to enhance dissemination efforts. A quick online search reveals the breadth of existing infographics across public health topics.

There are many ways to create an infographic for specific study data using existing templates and resources. There are software programs dedicated to the creation of infographics, varying in their capabilities and ease of use. Some programs and templates are free, others require program or subscription purchase. Many are easy to use even without a background in graphic design. The overall goal of your message should guide decisions on what to include and how to format the information. Because there are almost endless choices in ways to depict data, it is helpful to develop several versions of an infographic and pilot test them for understandability and visual appeal with varied stakeholders. Use the pilot-test data to inform the final version. Another important consideration is developing the infographic in formats that can be easily shared through downloads or social media. This increases the reach and impact of public health research results.

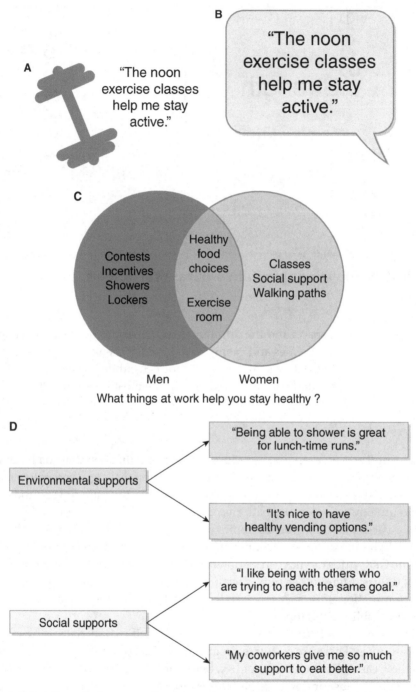

FIGURE 14.7 **Visualizing qualitative data with quotes. (A) Example of a quote and corresponding icon, (B) example of a quote in a callout box, (C) example of a Venn diagram, and (D) example of a concept map.**

EXHIBIT 14.2 EXAMPLE OF A CDC INFOGRAPHIC

The New (Ab)Normal

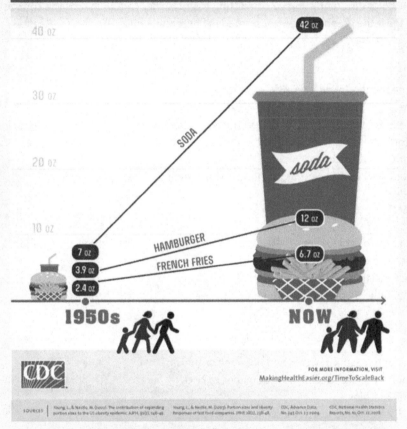

Source: Division of Nutrition, Physical Activity, and Obesity, National Center for Chronic Disease Prevention and Health Promotion. (2017). Centers for Disease Control and Prevention. Accessed November 5, 2019. https://www.cdc.gov/nccdphp/dnpao/multimedia/infographics/newabnormal.htm[5]

WHAT MAKES A GOOD CHART OR GRAPHIC?

Choosing the type of chart is only part of effective data visualization. Characteristics such as color, font, placement, and white space are also important to consider when preparing charts, graphs, or other visuals.

COLOR

- Objects or text that you wish to highlight should be in a color that contrasts with the background.
- Too many colors can be distracting. Try using different hues of the same color.
- Be consistent with color throughout the graphic.
- Use intuitive colors that match with the theme of the data.
- Consider the use of patterns to make the information readable to those who may be color-blind.
- Test the color differentiation by converting to grayscale. This will show the contrast within the image if the graphic is seen or printed in black and white.

FONT

- Limit the number of different types of font within the same graphic.
- Choose a typeface that works well in various sizes.
- Choose the proper font size based on the ways the graphic will be viewed. There are minimum font-size recommendations for phone screens, desktops, PowerPoint presentations, and printed material.
- Avoid using all caps in text blocks longer than one line.

PLACEMENT

- Organize elements to create vertical and horizontal lines throughout the graphic.
- Left justify the text.
- Be sure to align table/figure titles.
- Consider labeling figures so no legend is needed.

WHITE SPACE

- Leave adequate space within and between graphics.
- Maintain adequate spacing between lines of text.
- Maintain margins.
- Avoid the impulse to fill extra negative space.

CHAPTER DISCUSSION QUESTIONS

1. Give an example of a recent visualization of health data you saw in the media.
2. Why is data visualization important to public health research?
3. What are some challenges to presenting data through visualization effectively?
4. What factors should you consider when choosing the best type of data visualization?
5. How can infographics be used to increase the impact of public health research findings? Find an online example and critique it using information from this chapter.

RESEARCH PROJECT CHECK-IN

Your Creativity is Calling

Now that you have your results and conclusions from your study, it's time to develop effective ways to present it. There are many techniques you can use to depict your findings in graphics and other visualizations. The good news is that many of these strategies are built into commonly used statistical analysis software or other database programs. Because there are many ways to depict the same data, try a few of them, and pilot test them to see whether they convey the data in the way you intended. Try your hand at infographics. They are great for inclusion in many types of dissemination products.

PUBLIC HEALTH RESEARCH METHODS IN REAL LIFE

Visuals Worth a Thousand Words

The presentation was not well received. Jordan heard members of the audience saying things like, "I can't even read that small print!" or "What do those numbers even mean?" He even heard one person make a comment about the project being a waste of time and money. The purpose of this community forum was to present data and make recommendations for new food markets in area food deserts. The research team spent the last 6 months aggregating relevant sociodemographic data and collecting primary data using mixed methods. Community residents were heavily involved in the planning and implementation of this study. It was now very apparent that community members should have been involved in development of this presentation.

This was one of Jordan's favorite projects since becoming a research coordinator in the academic research center. His center partnered with local community agencies with the goal of improving health equity in the region. The impetus for this project was a federal report that identified metropolitan food deserts, or areas without adequate resources and access to fresh foods. Parker Heights, the area where the research center was located, had the highest number of food deserts in the whole state.

Jordan found different sources of national, state, and local data. He also collected information on how other similar regions were addressing this issue. He and the research team conducted community audits, key-informant interviews, and focus groups. He also led part of the project for which residents took pictures of things in their everyday lives that might impact food access. He will always remember the picture of the three bus stops one resident provided. For this resident, the nearest grocery store was three bus transfers away from his home.

They had a lot of data to present back to the community. The members of the research team knew how to write academic papers and reports but had little expertise in ways to visualize data that nonacademics would understand. It was easy to make tables and charts, and fill slides with words and numbers, so that is what they did for this community forum. The presentation included several data tables copied and pasted right from the census website. Audit data were presented in graphs with no data labels. Summaries of interview data were squeezed onto one slide. Another slide had five verbatim quotes from focus group participants. The presentation would have been fine for a public health conference presentation, but it wasn't effective in showcasing the food desert research to the community.

The principal investigator who was presenting at the forum didn't need to look at the evaluations to know it did not go well. The community residents seemed to be confused by the data and did not have the right information to make informed recommendations for prioritizing efforts to improve local food deserts. The research team decided to meet with community stakeholders and advisors to plan another forum. They decided to seek out someone at the university who could provide assistance in developing simple, yet effective visualizations of their data. They would use infographics and visual summaries instead of lots of numerical tables and charts. Perhaps the most important part of this redo would be planning and pilot testing the visualizations with community residents and advisors before presenting it.

After this experience, Jordan volunteered to take a course in data visualization. After seeing his colleagues struggle with this type of presentation, and watching the audience reaction at the food desert forum, he wanted to enhance his skill set and use the skills toward improving health equity through the research center, one visualization at a time.

Critical Thinking Questions

1. How can public health students and practitioners gain better skills in data visualization?
2. In what ways might data visualization be useful in presenting complex health information to varied audiences?
3. What are some disadvantages of using simple visualizations instead of presenting all the results?
4. Why should the visualizations for nonacademic audiences be created and tested with help from members of the target population? What might go wrong if this is not done?
5. Visualizations can be powerful for gaining support on a public health issue. What are some examples of data presented in a way that informed your opinion or influenced your support of an issue?

COUNCIL ON EDUCATION FOR PUBLIC HEALTH FOUNDATIONAL KNOWLEDGE AND COMPETENCIES

Foundational Knowledge

Profession and Science of Public Health

- Explain the critical importance of evidence in advancing public health knowledge.

Foundational Competencies

Evidence-Based Approaches to Public Health

- Interpret results of data analysis for public health research, policy, or practice.

Communication

- Communicate audience-appropriate public health content, both in writing and through oral presentation.
- Describe the importance of cultural competence in communicating public health content.

REFERENCES

1. Friendly MA. Brief history of data visualization. In: Chen C, Hardle W, Unwin A, eds. *The Handbook of Data Visualization*. New York, NY: Springer Publishing Company; 2008:16–48.

2. Kirk A. *Data Visualisation A Handbook for Data Driven Design*. Thousand Oaks, CA: Sage; 2016. Accessed November 1, 2019. https://us.sagepub.com/sites/default/files/upm-binaries/75674_Kirk_Data_Visualisation.pdf

3. Clark R, Lyons C. *Graphics for Learning*. 2nd ed. San Francisco, CA: Pfeiffer; 2011.

4. Centers for Disease Control and Prevention. FluVaxView: Estimates of influenza coverage among adults—United States, 2017–2018 flu season. 2018. Accessed November 5, 2019. https://www.cdc.gov/flu/fluvaxview/coverage-1718estimates.htm

5. Division of Nutrition, Physical Activity, and Obesity, National Center for Chronic Disease Prevention and Health Promotion. Centers for Disease Control and Prevention. 2017. https://www.cdc.gov/nccdphp/dnpao/multimedia/infographics/newabnormal.htm

6. Council on Education for Public Health. Accreditation Criteria: Schools of Public Health & Public Health Programs. 2016. Accessed September 7, 2019. https://media.ceph.org/wp_assets/2016.Criteria.pdf

ADDITIONAL READINGS AND RESOURCES

Centers for Disease Control and Prevention. Graphics and infographics. n.d. Updated October 21, 2016. Accessed November 5, 2019. https://www.cdc.gov/flu/resource-center/freeresources/graphics/index.htm

Evergreen SDH. *Effective Data Visualization: The Right Chart for the Right Data*. Thousand Oaks, CA: Sage; 2017.

Nussbaumer Knaflic C. *Storytelling with Data: A Data Visualization Guide for Business Professionals*. Hoboken, NJ: John Wiley & Sons; 2015.

Strecher V, Zikmund-Fisher BJ. Visualizing health: A scientifically vetted style guide for communicating health data. 2014. Accessed November 5, 2019. http://www.vizhealth.org

Disseminating Research Results

People hear statistics but they feel stories.
> —Brent Dykes, Senior Director of
> Data Strategy, DOMO

LEARNING OBJECTIVES

After reading this chapter, the reader will be able to

- Develop an effective dissemination plan.
- Understand the importance of the audience for dissemination efforts.
- Implement social math strategies for messaging.
- Define *health literacy*.
- Apply strategies to improve effectiveness of dissemination efforts.

INTRODUCTION

Public health research creates new knowledge, and sharing this knowledge with others is the final phase of the research process. After all, what good is research if no one knows about it? Disseminating results is a necessary step toward building evidence to impact public health practice and policy. The word disseminate stems for the Latin word *disseminare*, which means scattering seeds. Like seeds, research results can be widely dispersed to propagate evidence. In a research context, **dissemination** is a systematic, active approach of spreading research findings and evidence-based interventions to the target audience via determined channels using planned strategies.[1] Similar to dissemination, the term knowledge translation is also used to describe this important phase of the research process. Widely used outside of the United States, **knowledge translation** is defined as the synthesis, dissemination, exchange, and ethically sound application of knowledge to improve health.[2] Whatever term is used, planning and implementing strategies to share research findings should not be overlooked.

Diffusion is another term used to describe the way in which research results are distributed. **Diffusion** refers to passive, untargeted, unplanned, and uncontrolled spread of a new intervention or idea.[1] Think about how new trends start. If a famous celebrity wears a certain bracelet, maybe the popularity of that bracelet spreads widely. In many cases like the bracelet example, there was no plan for the way the popularity diffused. It just happened. Dissemination is not passive or spontaneous. It is an active or purposeful approach and must be deliberate and systematic to be effective. If we waited for diffusion to occur, it might never happen or take years to understand and apply evidence-based public health practices and policies.

SCURVY AND SLOW DISSEMINATION

James Lind was a Scottish naval surgeon in the mid-18th century. On long voyages at sea, Dr. Lind saw the devastation caused by scurvy. Those inflicted had debilitating symptoms and often died. In 1747, Lind conducted what is known as the first randomized control trial to figure out the most effective way of treating and preventing this illness. Of the several strategies Lind used, citrus juice proved to be the best treatment. Six years later, he published "A Treatise of the Scurvy" describing his research results. It was not until 1795 that Lind's findings were put into practice. Almost 50 years after the original experiment, the Royal Navy adopted the practice of supplying lemon juice on ships to prevent scurvy.[3] Think of how many lives could have been saved during those 50 years if Lind had planned and implemented a good dissemination plan!

CHALLENGES TO DISSEMINATION

The need for better dissemination in public health is well established.[4] Billions of dollars are spent on the development of interventions to prevent disease and promote health, but few are translated into practice. Most public health researchers understand its important role in research, but they dedicate little time to the dissemination process.[4] There are several reasons for this disconnect. The first has to do with priorities in academic research. Researchers often prioritize sharing findings solely with other researchers. Peer-reviewed papers have the most career impact for academic researchers, but results published in academic journals are not likely to reach other important audiences. Accessing the papers can be difficult and costly outside of the research world. The papers are also written in ways that researchers can understand and replicate, but this makes it difficult for other stakeholders or the public to comprehend the study results.

Lack of knowledge and skills is another reason for poor dissemination. Most researchers are very good at academic writing, but find it difficult to translate complex studies or complicated results in language the general population will understand. Without dissemination knowledge and skills, communicating results beyond the research world is unlikely to happen. Fortunately, the upcoming generation of public health researchers will be better equipped to plan and implement dissemination strategies. The updated foundational competencies required by the Council on Education for Public Health include a category for learning to effectively communicate health content to a wide variety of audiences. All students in accredited public health schools and programs should be gaining skills to make dissemination a standard practice in research. In addition to formally acquiring skills, we can also learn a great deal about dissemination from the populations we study. Public health researchers should engage with the community or be advised by relevant stakeholders throughout the research process, but this collaboration is especially important during the dissemination phase. By doing this, researchers can not only learn what content is most important to share, but also the most effective means to getting the information to them.

Another challenge to dissemination is timing. Dissemination is the last phase in the research process. As mentioned previously in this book, unanticipated factors may extend the time it takes to conduct research studies. Maybe you planned for 3 months to prepare and disseminate findings to various audiences, but recruitment of participants took longer than expected or there were problems with the data and several analyses had to be conducted and you barely had enough time to complete the study in the time allowed by the funding agency. Timeline pressure and the end of grant funding can contribute to cutting corners when it comes to dissemination. Peer-reviewed papers and conference presentations are often the only products to evolve from studies due to lack of time.

Cost can be another barrier to dissemination efforts. Open-access publishing increases the breadth of disseminating research results, but also increases the cost of dissemination efforts. Open-access journal articles are those that do not require an association membership or fee in order to access them. If you are not a member of the American Public Health Association (APHA) or do not have access to an academic library subscribing to APHA's affiliated journal (American Journal of Public Health), the article would cost $24 to download. If it was an open-access article, the article would be free to anyone. Although free to the public, open-access comes at a cost to the researcher. The cost to the researcher varies by the type of article and journal, but it can range from hundreds to thousands of dollars to publish an open-access peer-reviewed paper. For example, the 2020 open-access fee for the American Journal of Public Health was $2,500. The fees go to processing the article and maintaining it for access in the system. Many researchers are opting for open access and build the cost into grant-proposal budgets. But as these open-access fees rise, some funders are capping the allowable amounts for open-access publishing. It is important to note that all papers from National Institutes of Health-funded research must be made available to the public within 12 months of publication through PubMed Central, a publicly accessible digital archive (http://www .ncbi.nlm.nih.gov/pmc). There is no fee to the researcher to contribute to this archive, and it is required by law.

Public health researchers can disseminate results to other researchers through presentations at professional conferences or other meeting venues. However, conference fees, travel, lodging, and transportation costs can stretch budgets. The fee just to attend the National Conference of the American Public Health Association in 2020 was $600, not including annual membership dues. It is not just papers and conferences that are cost barriers. Translating research findings to reach nonacademic audiences comes with a price, too. If a research team lacks expertise, it can be costly to hire consultants who specialize in things like data visualization or media communication.

These challenges to dissemination are not insurmountable. Several main funders of public health research now require a dissemination plan as part of grant applications. These requirements help researchers prepare for dissemination early in the research process, including building it into project timelines and budgets. In addition, requiring a dissemination plan holds researchers accountable to implement the plan if they are granted research funds. Technological advancements (e.g., online analytics)also facilitate research dissemination. Integrating metrics into peer-reviewed papers (see Figure 15.1 for an example) helps publicize the extent to which research findings are disseminated beyond the journal article. Altmetrics is one product to track and visualize the reach and influence of research.[5] This application is a collated record of all online shares and mentions of the research visualized to show various dissemination outlets of published content. Analytics, such as Altmetrics, are becoming increasingly popular as part of overall dissemination strategies among researchers.

PLANNING FOR DISSEMINATION

Even though dissemination is the last phase of the research process, plans for sharing results should be built into the early stages of a research study. A dissemination plan defines who your audience is and how best to reach them for maximum impact. Plans also help identify the structure for distributing results and messages, along with the timing and type of delivery. Good plans also include identification of who will be responsible for the outlined strategies. Research team members can prepare for their dissemination role during the phases of the research process.

Many theoretical dissemination frameworks and models have been developed to help facilitate the transfer of research knowledge into practice and policy. For example,

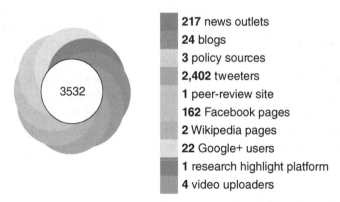

217 news outlets
24 blogs
3 policy sources
2,402 tweeters
1 peer-review site
162 Facebook pages
2 Wikipedia pages
22 Google+ users
1 research highlight platform
4 video uploaders

3532

FIGURE 15.1 Example of a metric summarizing dissemination of an academic paper.

Source: Courtesy of Altmetric.

interest in identifying dissemination best practices led to the creation of the Designing for Dissemination, Implementation, and Sustainability (D4DIS) framework. D4DIS refers to a set of recommended processes and activities that are performed during planning, development, and evaluation of an intervention to maximize dissemination potential.[6,7] This framework is based on key principles such as:

- Dissemination should be an active and systematic approach.
- Dissemination should be planned early in research phases.
- Researchers should partner with target users to enhance effectiveness of dissemination efforts.
- It is essential to know and understand audience needs.

This framework can be a useful guide for creating and implementing a dissemination plan within public health research studies. In addition to the framework, there are many dissemination-plan templates available to guide planning. These templates provide a structure for identifying target audiences along with products and the medium by which to deliver them. Templates also include a place for identifying a timeline for planned dissemination products as well as the project personnel responsible. See Table 15.1 for a sample dissemination-plan template.

As mentioned previously, dissemination should be planned and purposeful. Many complex elements of public health research need to be carefully considered for dissemination strategies to be most effective.

TABLE 15.1 EXAMPLE OF A DISSEMINATION-PLANNING TABLE

Audience	Product	Medium	Release Date	Person Responsible	Follow-Up Notes
State policy makers	One-page summary	Print	November 2020	Staff A	Provide before press conference
Community members	Slide presentation	Verbal presentation at council meeting	January 2021	Staffs A and B	Mr. X will preview slides in December
Researchers	Manuscript	Print	November 2020	Staff B	Target journal is *AJPH*
Public	Social media post	Internet	February 2021	Staff A	Follow-up with most relevant outlets

1. **Goals for Dissemination.** Your research question provides a focus for your study throughout the research process. In the same way, dissemination goals provide the foundation for the ways in which you share results. Goals are at the heart of the dissemination plan because they outline the intended impact of dissemination efforts. Examples of dissemination goals include
   - Raise awareness about an issue.
   - Change practice.
   - Gain support for a policy or initiative.
   - Increase understanding.
   - Promote evidence.

   For example, suppose you conduct an environmental health study on the impact of noise pollution on children in a school near a construction site. Your dissemination goal might include changes in regulations about acceptable noise levels. This goal provides the hub on which to focus dissemination efforts.

2. **Audience.** A good dissemination plan anticipates groups interested in learning about study findings and those most impacted by the research results. The most relevant groups are directly related to the overall dissemination goals. For example, if a study provides information to support a new policy or initiative, policy makers would be a likely target audience. Perhaps the same study would also be of interest to community members who would be impacted by policy change. Results from an intervention study might add new evidence to a health topic, and thus dissemination might be geared toward an academic research audience. Having multiple target groups in the dissemination plan may require various materials and strategies for distribution. **Audience segmentation** is the process of distinguishing among different subgroups of users and creating targeted marketing and distribution strategies for each subgroup.[7] Audience segmentation should be based on an understanding of subgroup information needs and preferences. The best way to gain this understanding is by partnering with representatives from each group. As indicated in the D4DIS framework, partnering with target users early in the development process can increase the success for later dissemination and implementation efforts.[4,6,8] Audience segmentation also encompasses learning about each target group. Researchers should investigate group priorities and audience perception of the issues being studied when planning for dissemination. It is also important to know what kind of information they need. For example, researchers might need statistical significance and methodological details, but city administration might need to know local relevance. This information will help make dissemination products more applicable and relevant to each group.

3. **Products and Outlets.** Another part of dissemination planning is knowing the specifics on where, when, and how target groups seek information. Not all groups will find a peer-reviewed manuscript useful. In fact, there is often a difference between what researchers think is the most relevant way to share findings, and what practitioners, community members, or policy makers actually find useful.[9,10] Partnering with members of groups informs the most relevant ways to reach each target audience. See Exhibit 15.1 for examples of two forms of dissemination of the same study information. This exhibit

shows a peer-reviewed paper from a study on how buildings influence physical activity. The same results were presented to building residents in a research brief. Both products present the same information, but do so in different ways for different audiences. Some common dissemination products are:

- **Peer-reviewed manuscripts** are a standard way to reach an academic audience. Journals can be content specific (e.g., *Preventing Chronic Disease*), method specific (e.g., *Qualitative Health Research*), or more general (e.g., *American Journal of Public Health*). These are formal, scientific outlets that are less accessible and less useful to audiences outside of research.
- **Conference presentations** are another way to reach an academic research audience. Most professional organizations host national or regional meetings where researchers can showcase their work. Conference presentations typically come in two formats. Oral presentations are classic presentations in front of an audience and poster presentations are visual summaries displayed for attendees during conferences. Conference presentation abstracts are also summarized and published in conference proceedings so even nonattendees can access the information.
- **Research briefs and reports** are shorter and less formal than peer-reviewed articles. In these documents, text is usually enhanced with data visualization and infographics. These depict main findings, succinct results, and often include recommended actions or next steps. There is no consensus on the most effective attributes to use, and length and structure of research briefs vary tremendously.
- **Presentations to stakeholder groups or community members** can be an effective way to maintain partnerships and support research. These presentations provide a good venue for clarification and feedback from people impacted by the results. Understanding group priorities, perceptions, and needs is vital for the success of these presentations.
- **Workshops and seminars** are a good way to reach practice audiences. Many professional groups or associations have existing mechanisms by which they provide trainings. Partnering with these groups can enhance reach and impact. For example, the National Association for Chronic Disease Directors (NACDD) hosts events such as regular member webinars and highlights relevant research on its website.
- **Social media posts** are emerging as an effective way to reach different audiences, but are only utilized by a small percentage of health researchers.[11] Formats vary by social media outlet, and range from brief statements, to links, to full reports or academic papers. More research is needed to add to the emerging evidence on the effectiveness of specific social media dissemination strategies.

The dissemination plan should also outline how the products are delivered. The internet allows for inexpensive and easy ways to disseminate research results through email, websites, and social media. Webinars are another way to reach many people without the inconvenience and cost of travel to face-to-face trainings. Research results can also be distributed through more traditional mass-media outlets such as newspapers, radio, and television. Other options include mailings or in-person distribution of printed research information. Several factors should go into choosing delivery strategies. These include preference of group, feasibility of method, timeliness, cost, and contribution to the overall dissemination goal.

4. **Execution.** A proposed timeline of activities facilitates effective execution of the dissemination plan. Past experiences and partnerships can provide estimates of how long the dissemination strategies might take. Keep in mind, though, that some strategies take longer than others. Publishing a peer-reviewed paper can take 6 to 12 months. There may be opportunities throughout the early steps of the research process during which information can be shared. For example, specific research methods or pilot results may be of interest to some audiences. In addition to specifying the timeline, clarifying who is responsible for execution of the different components of the dissemination plan increases accountability and likelihood for successful execution.

5. **Evaluation.** How will you know whether you met your dissemination goals? Evaluation strategies can quantify success in sharing research results to target audiences and can assess the way they used the information. Data from evaluation of dissemination strategies are also useful to show funders or other stakeholders the reach and impact of your work. For information shared online, technology has made it easy to collect, measure, and analyze Internet data. For example, downloads, views, and average length of time spent looking at a webpage can be informative analytics. Tracking citations from published work is a way to assess reach to the academic research audience. You can also incorporate postdissemination surveys or interviews to learn more about the perception and influence of the work from different groups.

EXHIBIT 15.1 EXAMPLES OF TWO DISSEMINATION PRODUCTS OF RESULTS FROM THE SAME STUDY

A. A peer-reviewed paper in a journal appropriate for the study topic

Journal of Physical Activity and Health, 2018, 15, 355-360
https://doi.org/10.1123/jpah.2017-0319
© 2018 Human Kinetics, Inc.

Human Kinetics
ORIGINAL RESEARCH

Can Building Design Impact Physical Activity? A Natural Experiment

Amy A. Eyler, Aaron Hipp, Cheryl Ann Valko, Ramya Ramadas, and Marissa Zwald

Background: Workplace design can impact workday physical activity (PA) and sedentary time. The purpose of this study was to evaluate PA behavior among university employees before and after moving into a new building. **Methods:** A pre–post, experimental versus control group study design was used. PA data were collected using surveys and accelerometers from university faculty and staff. Accelerometry was used to compare those moving into the new building (MOVERS) and those remaining in existing buildings (NONMOVERS) and from a control group (CONTROLS). **Results:** Survey results showed increased self-reported PA for MOVERS and NONMOVERS. All 3 groups significantly increased in objectively collected daily energy expenditure and steps per day. The greatest steps per day increase was in CONTROLS (29.8%) compared with MOVERS (27.5%) and NONMOVERS (15.9%), but there were no significant differences between groups at pretest or posttest. **Conclusions:** Self-reported and objectively measured PA increased from pretest to posttest in all groups; thus, the increase cannot be attributed to the new building. Confounding factors may include contamination bias due to proximity of control site to experimental site and introduction of a university PA tracking contest during postdata collection. Methodology and results can inform future studies on best design practices for increasing PA.

Keywords: evaluation, accelerometry, built environment

(continued)

EXHIBIT 15.1 EXAMPLES OF TWO DISSEMINATION PRODUCTS OF RESULTS FROM THE SAME STUDY (*continued*)

B. A research brief/infographic distributed to the participants and stakeholders

HEALTHY HILLMAN
Brown Expansion Evaluation Project Results

Most adults spend an average of 2400 hours per year at work. The work environment contains opportunities to promote health, wellbeing, and collaboration while also contributing to environmental, social, and economic sustainability.

Background

In 2008, the Brown School at Washington University in St. Louis (WUSTL) began a new program in public health, substantially increasing the number of faculty and staff. Plans for a new, innovative building to accommodate this growth soon began. Researchers at WUSTL recognized the potential for a "natural experiment," to explore the impact of building design before and after the occupation of the new building through the Building Expansion Evaluation Project. In 2015, Hillman Hall opened adjacent to the existing buildings, Brown and Goldfarb Halls.

The Study

We studied three groups of faculty and staff at WUSTL before (Spring 2014) and after (Spring 2015) the completion of Hillman to measure physical activity, collaboration and sustainability:
- Movers - People who moved into Hillman
- Non-Movers - People who remained in Brown or Goldfarb
- Controls - People who worked at Sam Fox School of Architecture and Design

A wide variety of methods were used for data collection:
- Activity Monitors   - Text Messages
- Interviews   - Social Network
- Surveys   - Observations

Hillman's Healthy Features

Hillman contains many features that promote physical activity, collaboration, and sustainability.

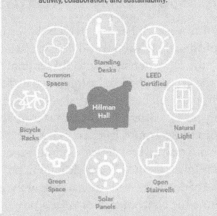

Common Spaces · Standing Desks · LEED Certified · Bicycle Racks · Hillman Hall · Natural Light · Green Space · Solar Panels · Open Stairwells

Physical Activity

Average Steps Per Week Increased in All Three Groups

Physical activity levels were consistent between accelerometer and self-reported survey data. The addition of Hillman, a new building and destination, increased steps for all groups.

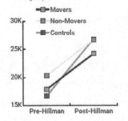

Pre-Hillman   Post-Hillman

Movers · Non-Movers · Controls

"I have a stand-up desk and I have yet to put it down. That doesn't mean I don't sit. I love having that standing desk."

Hillman & Brown/Goldfarb Occupants Feel More Supported to Exercise During the Workday

Movers and non-movers were more likely to feel supported than controls if they chose to exercise during the workday.

Hillman Occupants Move More
% of times moving in past hour by building.

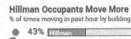
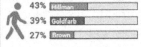

43% Hillman
39% Goldfarb
27% Brown

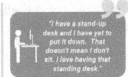

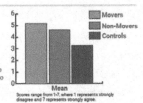

Mean
Scores range from 1-7, where 1 represents strongly disagree and 7 represents strongly agree.

Movers · Non-Movers · Controls

Sources: (A) Reproduced with permission from Eyler AA, Hipp A, Valko CA, et al. Can building design impact physical activity? A natural experiment. *J Phys Activ Health*. 2018;15:355–360. doi:10.1123/jpah.2017-0319;[12] (B) Courtesy of Amy Eyler.

An effective dissemination plan:

● Is built with partners, stakeholders, and end users.
● Includes a variety of dissemination methods and audiences.
● Leverages existing resources, relationships, and networks.
● Uses best practices for tailoring products and outlets to audience groups.
● Includes a well-developed evaluation plan for measuring reach and impact.

ETHICAL ISSUES RELATED TO DISSEMINATION

Public health research has the potential to influence population health and well-being, and because of this, there are ethical considerations when sharing results. As a researcher, you have the ethical responsibility to disseminate your results in ways that are accessible and useful to the groups likely to be impacted by the findings. One of the reasons vulnerable populations in particular may distrust researchers is because they have had experiences about which they never learned the outcomes from their contribution to the project. Reporting findings back to these groups is a necessary part of ethical dissemination.

There are also ethical considerations related to transparent and accurate reporting. Your work can inform the field of public health, but only if it is reported correctly with the appropriate level of detail. Presentation of research results should allow other researchers to be able to determine the contribution of your study to the overall evidence base. In the peer-review system used by academic journals, article reviewers are likely to point out any problems with the way the study was conducted or reported. In addition, many public health journals require authors to adhere to a code of ethics, which includes disclosure of contribution to the study, conflicts, funding sources, and honest reporting of results. See Exhibit 15.2 for information required by the *American Journal of Public Health* to ensure ethical and transparent research authorship.

The Equator Network: Enhancing the QUAlity and Transparency Of health Research
Enhancing the QUAlity and Transparency of Health Research is an international initiative that seeks to improve the reliability and value of published health research literature by promoting transparent and accurate reporting and wider use of robust reporting guidelines. It provides online resources for researchers and authors such as reporting guidelines, toolkits, and trainings. See https://www.equator-network.org for more information or to access helpful resources.

EXHIBIT 15.2 EXAMPLE OF AUTHOR ETHICAL RESPONSIBILITY AND DISCLOSURE IN PUBLISHING

The American Journal of Public Health
Authorship Criteria and Responsibility, Financial Disclosure, Copyright Transfer, and Acknowledgement and Informed Consent Statements

Each author (incl. corresponding author) must sign (1) the statement on authorship criteria and responsibility; (2) the statement on financial disclosure; and (3) either the statement of copyright transfer or the statement of federal employment. The corresponding author must sign (4) the acknowledgement and informed consent statement.

If necessary, copy and distribute or fax this form to your co-authors for their signatures. Signatures on one or multiple forms may be mailed to AJPH, 800 I St., NW, Washington, DC 20001-3710 or emailed to ajph.submissions@apha.org.

Corresponding Author's Name: _____   **Manuscript Number AJPH-** _____

Authorship Criteria and Responsibility. All authors certify that they meet the following criteria:

· Sufficient participation in the work to take public responsibility for the content.
· (1) Substantial contribution to the conception and design or analysis and interpretation of data, (2) drafting or revision of content, and (3) approval of the final version to be published.
· No prior publication of this manuscript or one with substantially similar content, except as described in the submission letter or here as an attachment.
· Willingness to provide data on which the manuscript is based for examination by the editors or their assignees.

Signature   Printed Name   Date Signed
_____
_____
_____
_____
_____
_____

Financial Disclosure. All authors certify disclosure of the following:

· All affiliations with or financial involvement with any organization or entity with a financial interest in the subject matter or materials discussed in the manuscript (e.g., consultancies, honoraria, stock ownership or options, expert testimony, grants, or patents received or pending, royalties) are disclosed in the submission letter or here as an attachment.
· All financial and material support for this work is clearly identified in the manuscript acknowledgment section.

Signature   Printed Name   Date Signed
_____
_____
_____
_____

Copyright Transfer. All authors must sign the following statement of copyright transfer or statement of federal employment below:

· In consideration of the action of the APHA in reviewing and editing this submission, the authors undersigned hereby transfer, assign, or otherwise convey all copyright ownership, including any and all rights incidental thereto, exclusively to the APHA, in the event that such work is published by the APHA.

Signature   Printed Name   Date Signed
_____
_____
_____
_____
_____

Federal Employment. I was an employee of the US federal government when this work was conducted and prepared for publication; therefore, it is not protected by the Copyright Act, and copyright ownership cannot be transferred.

Signature   Printed Name   Date Signed
_____
_____

Acknowledgment and Informed Consent. The corresponding author here certifies the following:

· All persons who have made substantial contributions to the work reported in this manuscript (e.g., data collection, writing, or editing) but who do not fulfill the authorship criteria are named in the acknowledgment section of the manuscript.
· Author has obtained (and will keep on file) all relevant consents for previously copyrighted photos/images (including photo subjects' consents) that will appear in the work.
· Absence of an acknowledgment section implies no other persons have made substantial contributions to this manuscript.
· All individuals specifically named in the acknowledgment section have provided written permission to be named.
· If human subjects are involved, approval by the institutional review board and the informed consent of participants has been obtained and reported in the acknowledgment section.
· Author acknowledges that APHA, as the publisher, has the right to make publication decisions regarding the work, including, without limitation, location of the work, timing of publication of the work, annotations and comments about the work, and the right to solicit opinions from others who may be interested in the subject matter of and opinions contained in the work.

Signature   Printed Name   Date Signed
_____

Source: Reproduced with permission from the American Journal of Public Health. American Public Health Association. *Guidelines for Authors.* 2020. Accessed November 12, 2019. https://ajph.aphapublications.org/page/authors.html

Researchers also have ethical responsibilities to those who provided the data and the groups they represent. As discussed in detail in Chapter 3, Ethics in Public Health Research, dissemination efforts need to uphold core ethical principles such as confidentiality and accurate representation. It is also essential to think about the potential outcomes of sharing results, and the impact this might have on these groups. Sometimes dissemination results in unanticipated consequences. Suppose your results show poor quality of fresh food in a local market. Stakeholders may use the report to demand better food choices from the vendor, but instead of making changes, the market closes, leaving behind a food desert for community residents. Knowing more about the community and developing relevant recommendations for next steps might have helped in this example. Although it is impossible to anticipate all unintended consequences, you can gain insight about the population and the context by involving community members and other stakeholders throughout the research process, including during dissemination.

Knowing and understanding the group's characteristics improves dissemination. Consider Internet access, for example. The level of Internet access within the target audience may impact the effectiveness of online information. Even with Internet access, consistency of service and technological skills are needed for online dissemination. Dissemination strategies should be tailored to meet the challenges of the target audience.

Literacy level of target groups is also a factor that is important to dissemination. According to the National Center for Education Statistics, 32 million American adults cannot read, and 50% of adults cannot read a book written at an eighth-grade level.[13] Low literacy levels result in limited ability to understand essential information, but there are strategies to address literacy concerns. Using plain language is one strategy for making written and oral information easier to understand.[14] Plain language documents are those in which users can find what they need, understand what they find, and act appropriately on that understanding. The U.S. Department of Health and Human Services provides resources and recommendations for improving the usability of health information, which are summarized in Table 15.2. There

TABLE 15.2 RECOMMENDATIONS FOR IMPROVING THE USABILITY OF HEALTH INFORMATION

Key Point	Strategies
Is the information appropriate for the users?	• Identify the intended user of the information. • Evaluate users' understanding before, during, and after the introduction of the information. • Acknowledge and respect cultural differences.
Is the information easy to use?	• Limit number of messages, use plain language, and focus on action. • Supplement with pictures. • Make written communication easy to read.
Are you speaking clearly and listening carefully?	• Check for understanding. • Use appropriate language.

Source: U.S. Department of Health and Human Services, Office of Health Promotion and Disease Prevention. Quick guide to health literacy. 2010. Accessed November 12, 2019. https://healthliteracycentre.eu/wp-content/uploads/2015/11/Quick-guide-to-health-literacy.pdf[16]

are also resources available to help develop documents within specific literacy parameters. The Flesch–Kincaid reading-grade level is designed to assess the difficulty in understanding text. Originally developed in 1948 by the Navy and Department of Defense, the formula factors in total words, total sentences, average sentence length, and average number of syllables per word. Scores range from low (0–30), indicating high difficulty best understood by college graduates, to high (90–100), which means the text is easily understood by the average 11-year-old/fifth grade student.[15] There are online versions of this formula, making calculation of reading level easy. Also, programs such as Microsoft Word have the capacity to calculate Flesch–Kincaid scores withingrammar review features. Consider literacy when developing dissemination materials to improve the likelihood your research results will be understood by the target audience.

TELLING THE RESEARCH STORY

Social Math

Disseminating data is only one aspect of facilitating awareness and understanding of research results. It is just as important to tell a compelling story with the data. Stories can help elicit action from the target audience, such as advocacy or policy support. Although there are volumes of textbooks and resources on communication and messaging through stories, several basic strategies can help improve public health research dissemination. The first is the concept of social math. **Social math** is the practice of making large numbers comprehensible and compelling by placing them in a context that provides meaning.[17] It is often difficult to judge the size or meaning of numbers without familiar or concrete comparisons. Think about the following fact from National Health Expenditure data:

> Out–of-pocket healthcare spending totaled $365.5 billion in 2017.[18]

It is difficult to comprehend the extent of $365.5 billion dollars, other than to realize the amount is *very large*. The long form of this number is $365,500,000,000! With social math, large numbers such as this can be described in ways that make more sense to the target audience. Extraordinarily large numbers can be presented in ways that make more sense to most people. For example, $365.5 billion can be translated to dollars per-person annual spending or divided and compared to some other type of purchase. The out-of-pocket spending amount could also be compared to total spending on food. There are many different ways to use social math to clarify public health research messages.[17]

1. Break the number down by time. If you know amounts per year, apply the data to smaller time frames such as per day or per hour. "There were 750,000 e-cigarettes sold in Monroe County this year. That's more than 2,000 per day in our small community."

2. Break the number down by place. Well-known places can help people understand the magnitude of the issue. "More than 30 million U.S. adults are now living with diabetes. That is equivalent to the entire population of Florida and Georgia combined."

3. Use local or personal comparisons. Make the data relevant by referencing local places or other comparisons based on the culture and context of the target audience.

"You could fill Busch Stadium at least 15 times with the number of people in St. Louis who don't have access to healthy food."

4. Use ironic comparisons. Point out skewed priorities by making unexpected comparisons. "Our survey found that 1,000 children in the Millersville school district are overweight or obese. That is 10X as many as the number of children enrolled in daily physical education."

Including social math as part of disseminating research messages can help make the results easier to understand and more memorable. Do some online searching on the ways social math is used for your topic of interest. These examples will be helpful in developing statements specific to your research findings. Report data in ways that are relevant to your target audience. It is also useful to pilot test the social math messages with representatives of target audiences to ensure understanding and relevance.

Single Overriding Communication Objective

Dissemination products vary in length and focus. Full-length manuscripts typically are between 3,000 and 5,000 words, whereas research briefs can consist of just 500 words. Social media posts are even shorter. For many audiences, succinct and focused messages are more effective than longer and more complex communications. One way to communicate your research story is to use the **single overriding communication objective (SOCO)** method. A SOCO is a key point or objective you want the audience to remember. It can also outline a call to action, as well as the benefit of taking action. Developing good SOCOs takes practice. It can be difficult to narrow down months (or years) of research into one objective. To develop a SOCO:

1. Write a short paragraph (four to five sentences or bullet points) to identify salient background information.
2. Write three to four facts or statistics you would like the target audience to remember about your story.
3. Define the primary and secondary populations you wish to reach.
4. Define the ONE message you want the audience to take away from this communication.

With a simple Internet search, there are many online resources and worksheets available to help you in the development of a SOCO. Work with research team members and others who might be experienced in SOCO messaging. Remember, it takes practice to boil down research information into this type of message, but SOCOs are a useful component of dissemination strategies.

BEST PRACTICES FOR EFFECTIVE DISSEMINATION

- Involve key stakeholders in planning dissemination.
- Make the ways to communicate research findings relevant to the audience.
- Be concise in messaging.
- Highlight key points to grab audience focus.
- Include graphics to break up text.
- Report recommended action.
- Evaluate and report dissemination impact.

CHAPTER DISCUSSION QUESTIONS

1. What system or policy-level changes could reduce the challenges to dissemination in public health research?
2. Describe an example of a research study in which the ethical implications of dissemination might be especially important.
3. How can you ensure research findings are presented with the appropriate literacy level and cultural context of the target population?
4. What audience characteristics might influence the impact of dissemination efforts?

RESEARCH PROJECT CHECK-IN

Get the Word Out

You have reached the final step in the research process. Congratulations! Research findings are used to build evidence and can change practice or policies only if people know about them. Plan your dissemination efforts to reach a broad audience. Tailor the products by target group, being sensitive to characteristics, culture, or preference. Don't underestimate the power of the SOCO. A simple, yet strong message about the results of your study can be an effective tool in increasing knowledge and support for important public health issues.

PUBLIC HEALTH RESEARCH METHODS IN REAL LIFE

Did You Read the Report I Sent?

Lois waited for the call or email from the school district superintendent about an endorsement of the new campaign to promote human papillomavirus (HPV) vaccines in school clinics. She knew the superintendent quite well and was confident he would support these efforts. She sent information to him last week with local data on HPV and HPV vaccine uptake. The report also included a cost-benefit analysis of providing the vaccine free of charge for students in the district. At the last minute she also decided to include some anecdotes from parents about the convenience of the school clinics, especially for well visits and vaccinations. The report she sent was about 10 pages long.

Her job as coordinator of school health practice at the local health department consisted of many duties. She often had to do site visits and meet with teachers and school nurses about different health issues. As she walked from the parking lot into Reaves High School, Lois noticed the superintendent walking into the school, too. She caught up with him and asked, "Did you read the report on HPV vaccines

I sent to you?" He knew the report she was talking about and was honest in saying he thumbed through it but didn't have time to read it all. He reminded Lois he gets dozens of documents to read each day and the ones that will take dedicated time to read get pushed aside in favor of the quick, bullet-point summary documents. "Boil the information down to what you think I need to make an informed decision about supporting the school HPV vaccine efforts. Use bullet points and data presented in a way I can easily get the gist," he told her as he walked into the principal's office.

She remembered from her MPH classes that decision makers had different dissemination needs than other groups, but she was so focused on getting him all the information, she did not put those lessons into practice. Now the project timeline was extended because the potential endorsement was pushed back. They couldn't move forward without his support.

Lois reviewed the information she originally sent to the superintendent. She agreed with his sentiments about it being lengthy. She even got bored reading it. She decided to look to the literature for research on policy maker's preferences in terms of the type of information they get. She found several published studies indicating a combination of short stories of constituents and local data worked best to garner policy maker support on public health issues. Another study found that anything over one page of text was unlikely to be read by policy or decision makers. She decided to use this information to refine the report for the superintendent.

The goal length for the revised report was one side of one page. Culling the 10 pages of text into this much shorter version would be quite a task. She recalled a time in her Epidemiology and Public Health Policy class when a state senator spoke as a guest speaker. Lois remembered the senator saying, "When you give me information, make sure it tells me the problem, options to fix it, and how much it will cost and/or save." She used these as the main headings for the report. She also added "the ask." Ultimately, she wanted the superintendent to publicly support the promotion of HPV vaccines in the school clinics. She clearly defined this request for the report. Instead of paragraphs of text, she included bullet points. She summarized the prevalence data in a chart and used data from other districts with similar programs to predict improvements. She also added an infographic that compared the cost of the vaccine per student with the cost of a pack of pencils. Last, she put in a quote from one of the parents in the district. It said, "I want to protect my child in any way I can, but I can't afford to take off work to get them to the doctor for the vaccine, especially when they would have to go more than once."

She had a few colleagues review the revised report and make suggestions for edits. She also showed her dad, who was a retired city administrator. He liked the way the information was presented and said he would endorse the program if it was up to him. He especially appreciated the short, easy-to-read-and-understand information.

Lois received a call from the superintendent 1 day after she sent him the report. He would endorse the program and formalize his endorsement in a written acknowledgment. He also told Lois she did a great job presenting 10 pages worth of information in one single page. He read the whole thing.

Critical Thinking Questions

1. How would a dissemination plan have helped Lois in this project?
2. What are ways to increase skills in effectively summarizing information for audiences such as policy makers?
3. Lois looked to the literature for information and evidence on best practices. What other resources could she have used in this quest?
4. What are some disadvantages to reducing information into a single message?
5. Why is it important to create ways to disseminate public health research for various audiences? How can this help solve complex public health problems?

COUNCIL ON EDUCATION FOR PUBLIC HEALTH FOUNDATIONAL KNOWLEDGE AND COMPETENCIES

Foundational Knowledge

Profession and Science of Public Health

- Explain the critical importance of evidence in advancing public health knowledge.

Foundational Competencies

Evidence-Based Approaches to Public Health

- Interpret results of data analysis for public health research, policy, or practice.

Communication

- Communicate audience-appropriate public health content, both in writing and through oral presentation.
- Describe the importance of cultural competence in communicating public health content.

REFERENCES

1. Lomas J. Diffusion, dissemination, and implementation: who should do what? *Ann N Y Acad Sci.* 1993;703(1):226–237. doi:10.1111/j.1749-6632.1993.tb26351.x

2. Straus SE, Tetroe J, Graham I. Defining knowledge translation. *CMAJ.* 2009;181(3–4):165–168. doi:10.1503/cmaj.081229

3. Brown SR. *Scurvy: How a Surgeon, a Mariner, and a Gentleman Solved the Greatest Medical Mystery of the Age of Sail.* New York, NY: St. Martin's Press; 2005.

4. Brownson RC, Jacobs JA, Tabak RG, et al. Designing for dissemination among public health research-ers: findings from a national survey in the United States. *Am J Public Health.* 2013;103(9):1693–1699. doi:10.2105/AJPH.2012.301165

5. Altmetric. Altmetric for researchers. 2020. Accessed September 7, 2020. https://www.altmetric.com/

6. National Cancer Institute. Designing for Dissemination: Conference Summary Report. December 18, 2002. Accessed September 7, 2020. https://cancercontrol.cancer.gov/IS/pdfs/d4d_conf_sum_report.pdf

7. Rabin BA, Brownson RC. Terminology for dissemination and implementation research. In: Brownson RC, Colditz GA, Proctor EK, eds. *Dissemination and Implementation Research in Health*. New York, NY: Oxford University Press; 2018:19–45.

8. Owen N, Goode A, Sugiyama T, et al. Designing for dissemination in chronic disease prevention and management. In: Brownson RC, Colditz GA, Proctor EK, eds. *Dissemination and Implementation Research in Health*. New York, NY: Oxford University Press; 2017:107–119. doi:10.1093/oso/9780190683214.003.0007

9. Brownson RC, Jones E. Bridging the gap: translating research into policy and practice. *Prev Med (Baltim)*. 2009;49(4):313–315. doi:10.1016/j.ypmed.2009.06.008

10. Brownson RC, Royer C, Ewing R, et al. Researchers and policymakers: travelers in parallel universes. *Am J Prev Med*. 2006;30(2):164–172. doi:10.1016/j.amepre.2005.10.004

11. Tunnecliff J, Ilic D, Morgan P, et al. The acceptability among health researchers and clinicians of social media to translate research evidence to clinical practice: mixed-methods survey and interview study. *J Med Internet Res*. 2015;17(5):e119.doi:10.2196/jmir.4347

12. Eyler AA, Hipp A, Valko CA, et al. Can building design impact physical activity? A natural experiment. *J Phys Act Health*. 2018;15:355–360. doi:10.1123/jpah.2017-0319

13. National Center for Education Statistics. National assessment of adult literacy (NAAL)—Demographics—Overall. 2010. Accessed November 12, 2019. https://nces.ed.gov/naal/kf_demographics.asp#3

14. U.S. Department of Health and Human Services. Health literacy—fact sheet: health literacy basics. Health communication. 2019. Accessed November 12, 2019. https://health.gov/communication/literacy/quickguide/factsbasic.htm

15. Kincaid JP, Fishburne Jr RP, Rogers RL, Chissom BS. Derivation of new readability formulas (automated readability index, fog count and Flesch reading ease formula) for Navy enlisted personnel. *Institute for Simulation and Training*. 1975;56. Accessed November 12, 2019. https://stars.library.ucf.edu/istlibrary/56/

16. U.S. Department of Health and Human Services, Office of Health Promotion and Disease Prevention. Quick guide to health literacy. 2010. Accessed November 12, 2019. https://healthliteracy-centre.eu/wp-content/uploads/2015/11/Quickguide-to-health-literacy.pdf

17. Berkeley Media Studies Group. Using social math to support your policy issue. 2015. Accessed November 11, 2019. http://www.bmsg.org/blog/using-social-math-to-support-your-policy-issue

18. Centers for Medicare and Medicaid Services. National Health Expenditure fact sheet—Centers for Medicare & Medicaid Services. 2018. Accessed November 11, 2019. https://www.cms.gov/research-statistics-data-and-systems/statistics-trends-and-reports/nationalhealthexpenddata/nhe-fact-sheet.html

ADDITIONAL READINGS AND RESOURCES

Berkeley Media Studies Group. Using Social Math to Support your Policy Issue. 2015. http://www.bmsg.org/blog/using-social-math-to-support-your-policy-issue/

Brownson RC, Eyler AA, Harris JK, Moore JB, Tabak RG. Getting the Word Out: New approaches for disseminating public health science. *J Public Health Manag Pract*. 2018; 24(2):102–111. doi: 10.1097/PHH.0000000000000673

Brownson RC, Colditz GA, Proctor EK, eds. *Dissemination and Implementation Research in Health: Translating Science to Practice*. 2nd ed. New York, NY: Oxford University Press; 2018.

Centers for Disease Control and Prevention. Sharing Health Literacy Research. 2018. https://www.cdc.gov/healthliteracy/disseminate.html

Centers for Disease Control and Prevention. Single Overriding Communication Objective Worksheet. Drinking Water Advisory Communication Toolbox. 2013. https://www.cdc.gov/tb/publications/guidestoolkits/forge/docs/13_samplesingleoverridingcommunicationsobjective_soco_work-sheet.doc

US Department of Health and Human Services, Office of Disease Prevention and Health Promotion. *National Action Plan to Improve Health Literacy*. Washington DC: 2010. https://health.gov/communication/hlactionplan/pdf/Health_Literacy_Action_Plan.pdf

Index